A **Foundation** COURSE IN
Child Care
& Education

Hodder & Stoughton

A MEMBER OF THE HODDER HEADLINE GROUP

Orders: please contact Bookpoint Ltd, 130 Milton Park, Abingdon, Oxon OX14 4SB. Telephone: (44) 01235 827720, Fax: (44) 01235 400454. Lines are open from 9.00–6.00, Monday to Saturday, with a 24 hour message answering service. Email address: orders@bookpoint.co.uk

British Library Cataloguing in Publication Data
A catalogue record for this title is available from The British Library

ISBN 0 340 801344

First published in 2001
Impression number 10 9 8 7 6 5 4 3 2 1
Year 2005 2004 2003 2002 2001

Typeset by J&L Composition Ltd, Filey, North Yorkshire
Printed in Italy for Hodder & Stoughton Educational, a division of Hodder Headline Plc, 338 Euston Road, London NW1 3BH.

Contents

Acknowledgements

Thank you to all those who kept saying 'Have you not finished that book yet?' without whom it may never have been completed.

Alison Mitchell

The authors and publishers would like to thank the publishers of *Nursery World* for allowing the reproduction of their cover. Thanks also to CACHE for use of materials on pages 32, 116 (kitchen illustration) and 150 (park illustration). All other illustrations were creat by Ian Foulis Associates and Chartwell Illustrators. Simon Cuerden took the photos on pages 57 (top) and 58 (top right).

The publishers would like to thank Gareth Thomas and Kay Guest at Campsbourne Junior School, London and Jon Goulding and staff at Campsbourne Infants for allowing us to take photographs and making us welcome. Many thanks to all the children who took part.

The publishers would like to acknowledge the following photographic agencies for permission to reproduce their images in this book:

Corbis: © Hans Georg Roth (p. 20); © Corbis/Reflections photo Library: Jennie Woodcock (p. 98 right)
Format: © Paula Bronstein (p. 13); © Paula Solloway (p. 19 left, p. 19 centre); © G. Montgomery (p. 19 right); © Joanne O'Brien (p. 23); © Jacky Chapman (p. 57 centre right); © Lisa Woollett (p. 59 bottom left and p. 83 bottom); © Judy Harrison (p. 62); © Sarita Sharma (p. 95); © Connie Treppe (p. 108)
PANews: © Haydn West (p. 11)
PhotoDisk: © Steve Mason (p. 57 bottom and p. 58 bottom right)
Photofusion: © Paul Baldesare (p. 16); © Crispin Hughes (p. 22); © Bipinchandra (p. 25); © Christa Stadtler (p. 54 left); © Paul Doyle (p. 54 centre); © David Montford (p. 54 right); © Ute Slaphake (p. 59 middle right); © Bob Watkins (p. 81); © Daliah Edwards (p. 121)

All other photographs were commissioned for this book and taken by **Gerald Sunderland.**

Introduction: Getting Ready to Study

This book has been written to help you learn more about caring for and working with young children.

There is a lot to learn but the information has been written in different ways, to help you understand and remember.

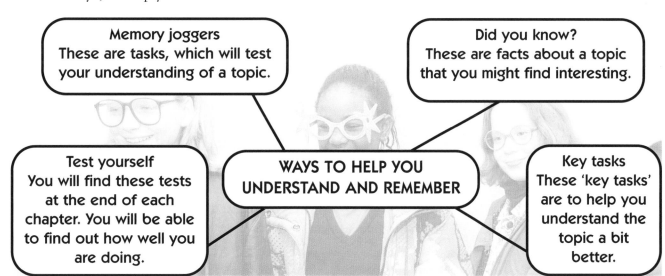

Memory joggers
These are tasks, which will test your understanding of a topic.

Did you know?
These are facts about a topic that you might find interesting.

Test yourself
You will find these tests at the end of each chapter. You will be able to find out how well you are doing.

WAYS TO HELP YOU UNDERSTAND AND REMEMBER

Key tasks
These 'key tasks' are to help you understand the topic a bit better.

FINDING INFORMATION

When you are working towards your qualification you will have to look for different kinds of information.

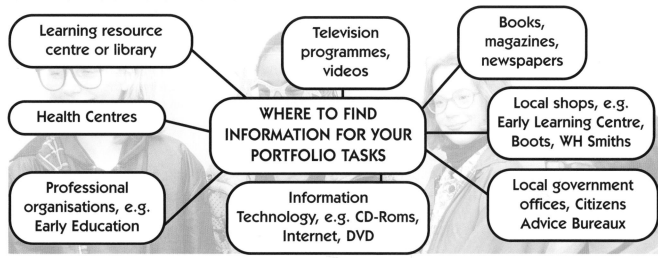

Learning resource centre or library

Television programmes, videos

Books, magazines, newspapers

Health Centres

WHERE TO FIND INFORMATION FOR YOUR PORTFOLIO TASKS

Local shops, e.g. Early Learning Centre, Boots, WH Smiths

Professional organisations, e.g. Early Education

Information Technology, e.g. CD-Roms, Internet, DVD

Local government offices, Citizens Advice Bureaux

Finding information in the learning resource centre

Sometimes it can be difficult to find information about child care in the learning resource centre because it is included in different sections.

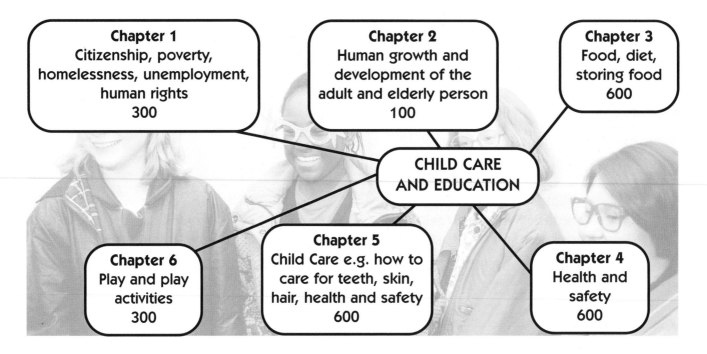

Chapter 1
Citizenship, poverty, homelessness, unemployment, human rights
300

Chapter 2
Human growth and development of the adult and elderly person
100

Chapter 3
Food, diet, storing food
600

CHILD CARE AND EDUCATION

Chapter 6
Play and play activities
300

Chapter 5
Child Care e.g. how to care for teeth, skin, hair, health and safety
600

Chapter 4
Health and safety
600

The number beside each subject tells you where to look for the book in the learning resource centre or library.

Magazines

There are different magazines you may find helpful when you prepare for your portfolio tasks, e.g. *Nursery World*, *Child Education*, *Parenting*.

KEY TASKS

Visit a local newsagent or shop that has a good selection of magazines. Ask the manager of the shop if you can make a list of the magazines that are about child care. **Remember that you can only read them if you are going to buy them.**

Finding information in books

When you begin the course, your tutor may suggest that you buy a particular book to help you. It is worth buying the book as you can then read it in your own time.

You may need to look at other books to give you more information.

Finding the right book

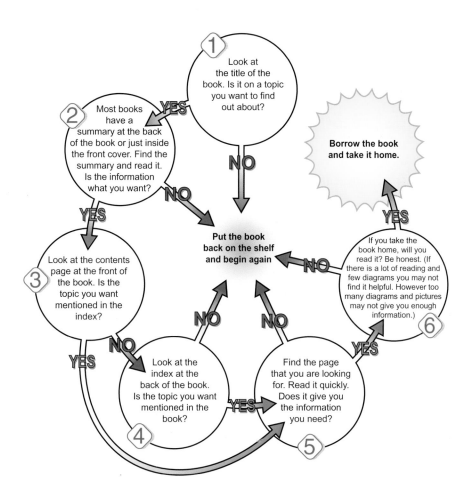

1 Look at the title of the book. Is it on a topic you want to find out about?

2 Most books have a summary at the back of the book or just inside the front cover. Find the summary and read it. Is the information what you want?

3 Look at the contents page at the front of the book. Is the topic you want mentioned in the index?

4 Look at the index at the back of the book. Is the topic you want mentioned in the book?

5 Find the page that you are looking for. Read it quickly. Does it give you the information you need?

6 If you take the book home, will you read it? Be honest. (If there is a lot of reading and few diagrams you may not find it helpful. However too many diagrams and pictures may not give you enough information.)

Borrow the book and take it home.

Put the book back on the shelf and begin again

Using the Internet to find information

If you want to find information quickly on the Internet it is useful to use a good search engine. One of the most powerful is *www.google.com*
All you need to do is enter the key words of the topic you are looking for and press enter. Do not include words such as 'and', 'the' or 'of'.
Throughout this book you will find web site addresses that will help you to gain more information about a particular subject.

Making a note of where you found the information

It is very important to make a list of where you found the information for your portfolio task. This is usually written in alphabetical order at the end of your piece of work.

If you used a book you need to give the information in the format shown below.

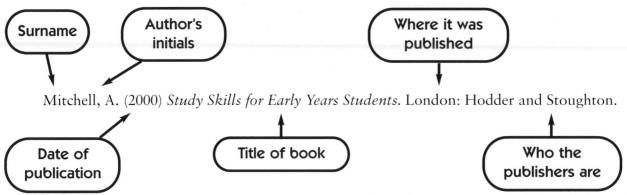

Mitchell, A. (2000) *Study Skills for Early Years Students*. London: Hodder and Stoughton.

If you use a magazine for information you need to give the author and date of publication, the title of the article and the name of the magazine.

Woolfson, R. (March 2001) 'They're off'. *Nursery World*.

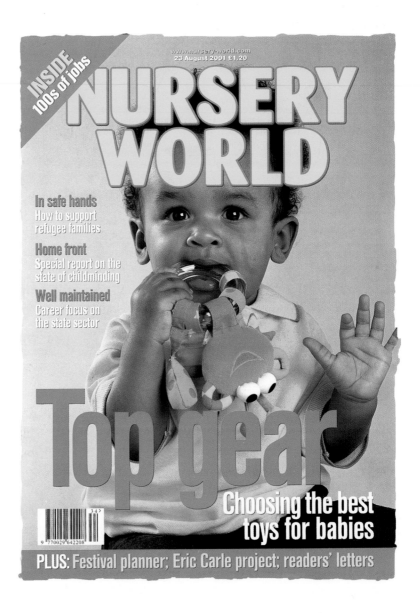

HOW TO USE THIS BOOK

This book is a source of information for your Foundation course. You can work your way through the book from page 1 to the end or you can dip in and out of it if you are looking for information on a specific topic.

Finding what you need

* The contents page at the beginning of the book will give you the title of the chapter and what it contains.
* Each chapter begins with bullet points, which tell you what information is going to be given.
* Each chapter has headings in large print which will help you to find the information quickly.
* There are Key Tasks boxes, Did You Know? and Memory Joggers to help you, and highlighted Key Words.
* The index at the back of the book gives you the page numbers for specific topics.

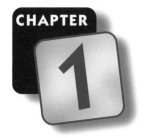

CHAPTER 1

Personal Development

* Being a responsible citizen
* Preparing for work
* Working effectively with others
* Working with children

1. BEING A RESPONSIBLE CITIZEN

What is a citizen?

There are different ways of becoming a legal citizen of a particular country. In Britain you are a British citizen if you have been born here or your parents are British citizens. You may have lived in another country and have applied to the government to become a British citizen.

As a British citizen, you have the right to:

* live in the UK,
* vote at elections and
* be protected by the law

You are expected to:

* obey the laws of the country
* pay taxes and
* respect the rights of others

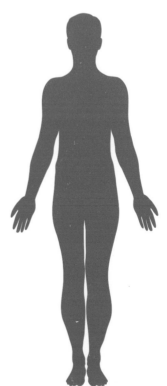

Who are good citizens?

What do you think makes a good citizen? Give as many reasons as you can.

Children from around the country were asked the same question. Here are some of their answers.

A good citizen cares and shares

A good citizen cares about the community and the world

A good citizen understands that rules are made for good reasons and does not break them

A good citizen respects people

KEY TASKS

Think of some famous people who you think are good citizens and give reasons for your answers.

Being a citizen within a community

Everyone belongs to different communities.

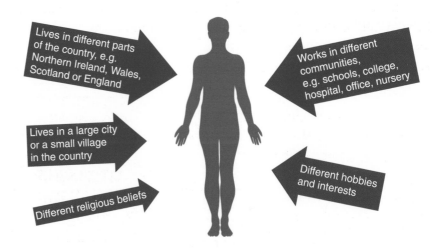

Lives in different parts of the country, e.g. Northern Ireland, Wales, Scotland or England

Works in different communities, e.g. schools, college, hospital, office, nursery

Lives in a large city or a small village in the country

Different hobbies and interests

Different religious beliefs

Some people feel a greater sense of belonging to their community than they do being a British citizen.

Being part of a community can affect your:

* behaviour
* language, dialect and accent
* independence, e.g. there are better transport systems in large towns and cities which allow you to go to different places more easily
* attitudes

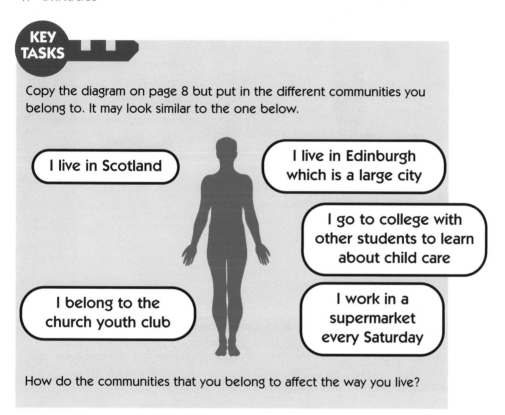

KEY TASKS

Copy the diagram on page 8 but put in the different communities you belong to. It may look similar to the one below.

I live in Scotland

I live in Edinburgh which is a large city

I go to college with other students to learn about child care

I belong to the church youth club

I work in a supermarket every Saturday

How do the communities that you belong to affect the way you live?

Citizenship education

Citizenship education has become part of the National Curriculum in England and Wales. Children study topics such as human and legal rights, voting, the role of the European Union and conflict situations.

For more information on citizenship access *www.citizen21.org.uk*

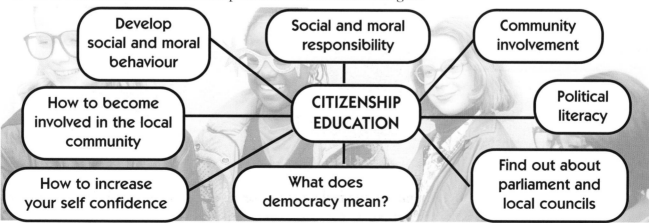

Develop social and moral behaviour

Social and moral responsibility

Community involvement

How to become involved in the local community

CITIZENSHIP EDUCATION

Political literacy

How to increase your self confidence

What does democracy mean?

Find out about parliament and local councils

How you can be a responsible citizen

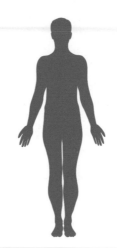

1. Know your rights and responsibilities and the rights of others

2. Care for others in the community

3. Care for the environment

4. Respect other people's religious beliefs, cultures and values

5. Have concern for people in other countries around the world and be aware of important issues throughout the world e.g. land rights

1. Know your rights and the rights of others

KEY TASKS

Do you think it is important to know your rights and responsibilities as a good citizen? Give reasons for your answer.

Every child and adult who lives in Britain has rights.

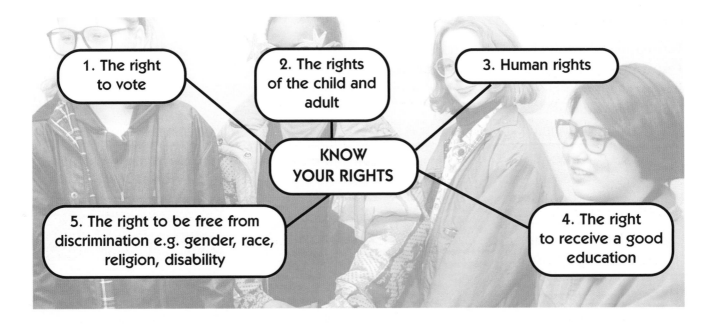

1. The right to vote

2. The rights of the child and adult

3. Human rights

KNOW YOUR RIGHTS

5. The right to be free from discrimination e.g. gender, race, religion, disability

4. The right to receive a good education

The right to vote

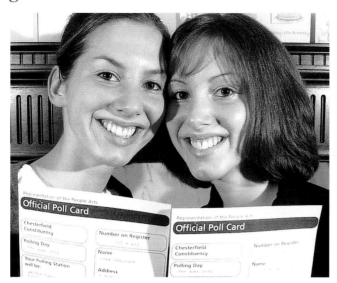

For most people, voting is the only way to have some influence over how the country is run. Most people over eighteen years of age have the right to vote.

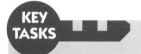

Why do you think only 12% of 18–24 year-olds vote in local council elections?

How people vote at a General Election

When there is a General Election, people living in the UK can vote for one Member of Parliament (MP) who is standing in a particular constituency (or area). The candidate with the most votes wins.

Scotland and Wales

In 1999, people living in Scotland voted for the first time for their own Scottish Parliament and people living in Wales voted for a Welsh Assembly. Each voter had two votes. One was for a Member of the Scottish Parliament or Welsh Assembly. The second vote was for a particular party.

European Elections

England, Wales, Scotland and Northern Ireland also have at the representatives European Parliament.

You must be registered on the **electoral role** before you can vote.

A card is sent to your house a few days before the election to tell you where and when you can vote.

On the day of the election, you take your card to the **polling station**.

Each ballot paper has a list of the candidate names on it and their parties. Beside each name is a box.

You will be given a **ballot paper** which you take to the **polling booth**.

When you go into the polling station you will be asked to give your name and they will tick it off their **electoral register**.

Read the ballot paper carefully and put **one** cross beside **one** name.

If you put more than one cross on the paper it becomes a **spoiled paper** and will not be counted.

When you have finished you fold the paper in half and put it in the ballot box.

You can post your vote if you are away from your home on the day of the election.

Your vote will now be counted along with everyone elses in that area and someone will be elected.

KEY TASKS

Do you think young people should be involved in the decision-making of the local community?

Discuss this topic with another person. You will need to decide before hand what you think about the topic and be able to speak clearly and answer questions.

The rights of the child and adult

Over the last few years a number of different laws have been introduced to protect the rights of children and adults.

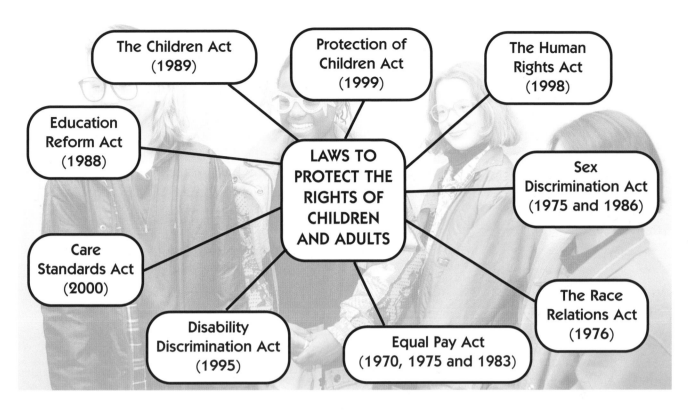

The Children Act (1989)

Protection of Children Act (1999)

The Human Rights Act (1998)

Education Reform Act (1988)

LAWS TO PROTECT THE RIGHTS OF CHILDREN AND ADULTS

Sex Discrimination Act (1975 and 1986)

Care Standards Act (2000)

The Race Relations Act (1976)

Disability Discrimination Act (1995)

Equal Pay Act (1970, 1975 and 1983)

The United Nations Convention on the Rights of the Child

Children have the right to be with their family or those who will care for them best.

Children have the right to enough food and clean water.

Children have the right to an adequate standard of living.

Disabled children have the right to special care and training.

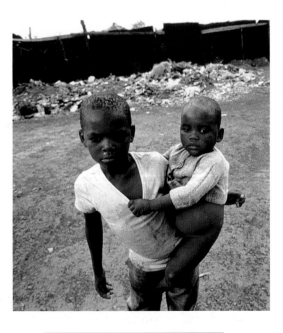

Children have the right to rehabilitation from cruelty, neglect and injustice.

Children have the right to health care.

Children have the right to be kept safe and not hurt, exploited or neglected.

Children must be allowed to speak their own language and practise their own religion and culture.

Children have the right to play.

Children have the right to free education.

Children have the right to express their own opinions and to meet together to express their views.

The Children Act (1989)

This Act is important because it states that children have rights and local authorities must ensure that the needs of the child are put first.

To protect children, the United Nations Conventions on the Rights of the Child was written. Britain agreed with the statements that were made and signed the agreement in 1991. The outline of The United Nations Convention on the Rights of the Child are on page 13.

Care Standards Act (2000)

This Act has changed the regulations for childminders and day care provision that were introduced in the Children Act 1998.

* A new early years department within OFSTED will inspect childminders and day care settings in England and Wales.
* Changes will be made to the Children Act.

Protection of Children Act (1999)

A list must be kept of people who are considered to be unsuitable to work with children.

The Human Rights Act (1998)

The Human Rights Act 1998 became law on 2 October 2000. If a person feels that their rights are being breached then they can take their case to a British court. Before this Act became law a person had to take their case to the European Court of Human Rights in Strasbourg.

People have the right:

* not to suffer degrading or inhuman treatment
* to a respect for private and family life, home and correspondence
* to freedom of thought, conscience and religious education
* to freedom of expression.

The Act applies to everyone within the UK, not just legal citizens but also temporary residents, e.g. asylum seekers.

Education Reform Act (1988)

All children in England and Wales must have access to the National Curriculum including children with special needs.

Sex Discrimination Act (1975 and 1986)

It is illegal for a person to refuse to give someone a job, buy or sell goods or prevent them from receiving an education because of their gender. It also protects people from sexual harassment.

Did you know?

In 1980 the Chinese government gave parents a higher salary, better housing and better education if they only had one child. What do you think about this?

Did you know?

Only about half the children in the third world get any formal education, and most of them leave before secondary school.

Disability Discrimination Act (1995)

This Act gives people who have a disability, new rights in relation to employment, access to facilities and services and buying and renting property.

Equal Pay Act (1970, 1975 and 1983)

Employers must pay the same for men and women if they are doing the same job.

To find out more about the National Minimum Wage you can look at *www.dti.gov.uk/er/nmw/*

The Race Relations Act (1976)

No one can discriminate (or treat differently) a person on the grounds of his/her race, ethnic or national origins, colour or nationality. It is illegal to refuse to give someone a job, buy or sell goods or prevent them from receiving an education because of their race.

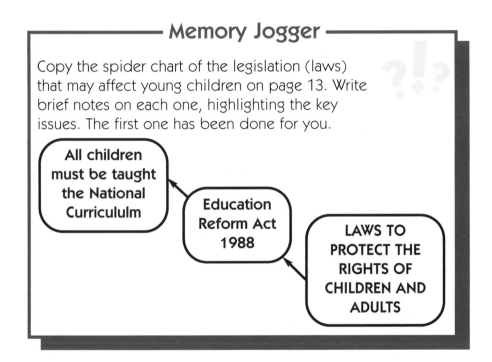

— Memory Jogger —

Copy the spider chart of the legislation (laws) that may affect young children on page 13. Write brief notes on each one, highlighting the key issues. The first one has been done for you.

All children must be taught the National Curricululm

Education Reform Act 1988

LAWS TO PROTECT THE RIGHTS OF CHILDREN AND ADULTS

2. Care for others in the community

Part of our responsibility as a member of a community is to be aware of and care for others.

We can care for others in our community in a number of different ways e.g. neighbourhood watch, doing tasks for neighbours who may not have the skills needed for the task, take part in local charity events.

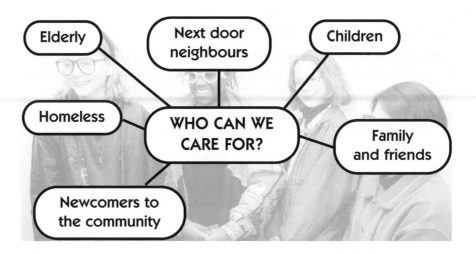

Elderly

Next door neighbours

Children

Homeless

WHO CAN WE CARE FOR?

Family and friends

Newcomers to the community

KEY TASKS

How can you care for others in your community? Think of a project that you could get involved in either on your own or as part of a small group. If possible, carry out your project. If you record what you have done in your project, you may be able to use the evidence towards your key skills portfolio.

KEY TASKS

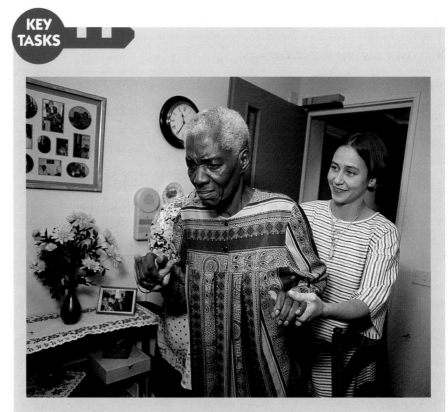

Look at the picture of the teenager above and answer these questions.

1 Describe what is happening in the picture.
2 How is citizenship being put into practice?
3 What can teenagers and elderly people gain from being together?

3. Care for the environment

Agricultural chemicals damage the soil and end up in our drinking water and the food we eat

Household and industrial waste is being dumped in landfill sites. This pollutes the soil.

Chemicals and untreated sewage has polluted the sea. This then affects the fish and other sea life.

WE ARE SLOWLY DESTROYING THE PLANET THAT WE LIVE ON.

There are approximately 500 different species of animal that are extinct. This has happened over the years because we have hunted them and destroyed the areas where they live.

We are polluting the atmosphere with fumes from car exhausts, factories and power stations.

The countryside is destroyed as more roads are built.

As good citizens, we have a responsibility to protect the environment for our own generation and future generations.

What can we do to help?

Recycling and reusing resources

✳ Reuse supermarket plastic carrier bags.
✳ Collect aluminium drink cans. You can get money for them.
✳ Use bottle banks, paper banks and clothes banks.
✳ Put labels on old envelopes and use them again.

Conserving energy

✳ Walk to college or take a bus instead of going by car.
✳ Switch off unwanted lights in the house.

Litter pollution

✳ Dispose of your litter carefully.
✳ Recycle or reuse it if possible.

Remember

✳ Broken glass, food tins and ring pulls cut animals and people.
✳ Plastic bags can suffocate.
✳ The faeces of animals can cause blindness in young children if they are in contact.
✳ Cigarette ends and matches cause fires.

Did you know?

Between 8 and 9 million disposable nappies are thrown away in the UK every day. It takes 50 to 100 years to decompose

Did you know?

America produces around 40 tonnes of solid waste per person each year

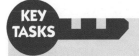

Design a poster that could be used in a childcare setting to encourage children and their parents to care for their environment.

4. Have concern for people in other countries around the world

The population of the world has increased rapidly over the last 300 years because:

* the death rate has dropped
* health care has improved over the last 100 years
* some life-threatening diseases no longer exist, e.g. smallpox
* fewer babies die in the first year of life
* people live longer.

However, difficulties arise as the population increases:

* there are housing shortages
* jobs are difficult to get
* more people move to the cities to try to find work
* in Third World countries babies and young children die of starvation and disease while other countries have too much food and waste it.

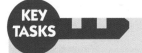

Find out about different organisations that care for other people throughout the world, e.g. the World Health Organisation (WHO) www.who.org World Food Programme www.wfp. org United Nations (UN) www.un.org

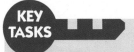

Work in a small group and talk about practical ways in which you could help other people in different countries throughout the world. If you have time and are interested, put your ideas into practice.

5. Respect other people's religious beliefs, cultures and values

Many different words are used when talking about the values in society today. It is important that you understand the differences

Prejudice
Attitudes or opinions about someone, which is not true but continued to believed even although they have not been proved

Cultural background
The beliefs and patterns of behaviour shown by a particular social group
A person's cultural background is shown in the way they speak, personal hygiene and daily routines
Each culture will have its own festivals and special occasions

Positive images
People and/or their cultures are shown in meaningful way, e.g. a woman as a firefighter

WHAT DO THESE WORDS MEAN?

Stereotype
Believe certain things about a group of people without knowing the true facts, e.g. All Eskimos live in igloos

Racism
The belief that one group of people is better that another

Role model
Someone who is a good example to others – the person may be from the same cultural group and of the same racial origin

Discrimination
Someone is treated less fairly than another person because he/she belongs to a particular group, e.g. racial discrimination, age discrimination

Racial awareness
Accepting and respecting the origins of people from different racial origins

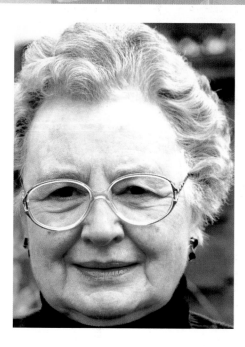
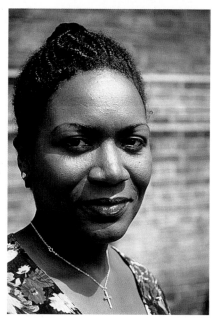
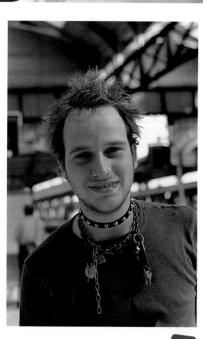

KEY TASKS

Look at the photographs on page 19 of a group of people.

① Who would you be most likely to share a personal problem with?
② What job (or not) do you think each of them has? Do you think anyone is unemployed?
③ Which person is most likely to have a drink or drug problem?
④ Who do you think is rich and who do you think is poor?
⑤ Who do you think is most likely to be violent?

Now talk about your answers in a small group.

✹ Do you show prejudice in any of your answers?
✹ Where do you think your prejudices come from?
✹ What can you do to change them?

Did you know?

Every day, about 16,000 new Christians are baptised in Africa.

Different religious beliefs

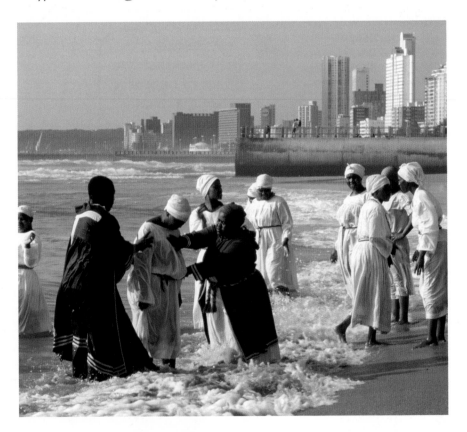

For many people, their religious belief is at the centre of their lives. It provides a guide to the way they live. Over three-quarters of the world's population is involved in different religions. You will learn more about different religious beliefs and the impact it can have on people's lives as you read through this book.

Equality of opportunity and anti-discriminatory practice

Equality of opportunity means:

✳ Treating children and adults equally according to their own needs. It does not mean treating everyone the same.

✳ Allowing everyone access to facilities, services, employment, etc. whatever their age, religion, race, culture, disability or gender.

KEY TASKS

'We are all different but we are all equal.' Talk about this statement in a small group. What do you think it means? How can you put it into practice when you are working with children?

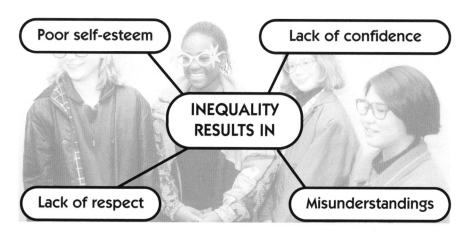

When working with young children we should:

✳ value their religious and cultural backgrounds
✳ value their disability, gender and life-style
✳ make sure that every child has the opportunity to join in
✳ understand that some children will be brought up to understand different values.

KEY TASKS

Watch two or three television advertisements. Do they promote equality of opportunity? Give reasons for your answers.

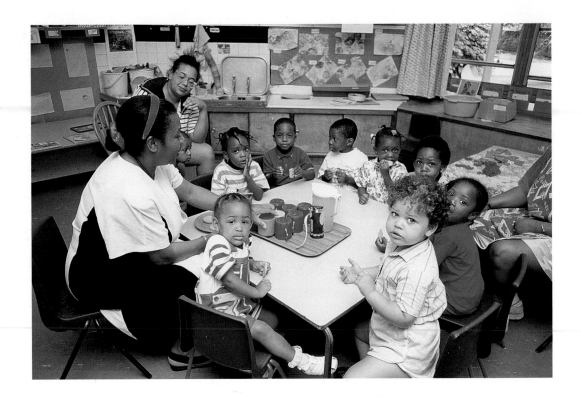

ENCOURAGING EQUALITY OF OPPORTUNITY IN THE CHILD CARE SETTING

✴ Find out about the different cultures that are represented in the child care setting. Talk to parents and other members of staff.

✴ Get to know every child's name as quickly as possible. Learn to pronounce them correctly.

✴ Find out about the different religious practices that the children in the work setting believe in.

✴ When you are preparing activities ask yourself, 'Can every child join in?', e.g., Can a child who is left-handed join in the cutting activities if there are only right-handed scissors?

✴ Be positive about every child. Do not make false assumptions about them.

Poverty

What does 'poverty' mean?

A couple with two children living on a family income of below £200 per week, after housing costs, would be living in poverty. A lone parent with one child would be living in poverty if they had a weekly income of below £105.

People who have low incomes find that they do not have enough money to buy essential items for an acceptable way of life. They are not able to join in the activities that are happening in their community. They can often feel left out.

The government help children and their families by giving money to those who need it, i.e. through benefits. Some families do not get these benefits and as a result they may find that they cannot pay for food, clothing or housing.

Children who are born into families experiencing poverty may find it hard to get out of the 'poverty trap'. They become trapped in the 'deprivation cycle'.

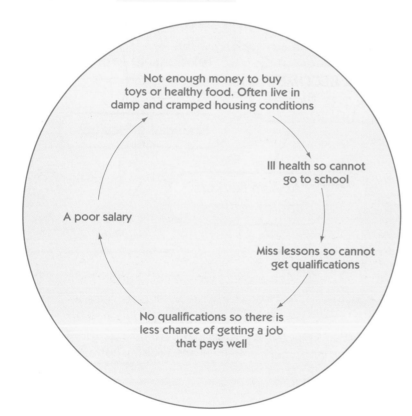

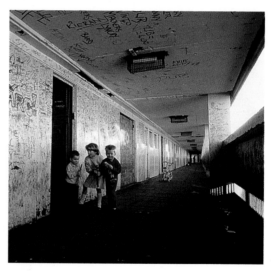

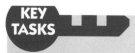

What effect could poverty have on a child?

Did you know?

A third of all children in the UK are living in poverty, i.e. approximately 4.4 million. A sixth of all children live in households where no one has paid employment.

40% of children live in the bottom 30% of the income distribution.

Homelessness

'Everyone has the right to a standard of living adequate for the health and well being of himself and of his family, including food, clothing and housing'.

United Nations Declaration on Human Rights

The number of homes in the UK rose by 50% between 1961 and 1997 and now totals 24,800,000. Approximately a quarter of these homes were built before the First World War and in some inner city areas this figure can be as high as 60%. Many of these homes are now in need of repair or demolition.

In the UK there are approximately 3 million people living in unsuitable conditions or are living 'on the street'. Worldwide there are approximately 150 million people living in unsuitable conditions.

Why do people become homeless in the UK?

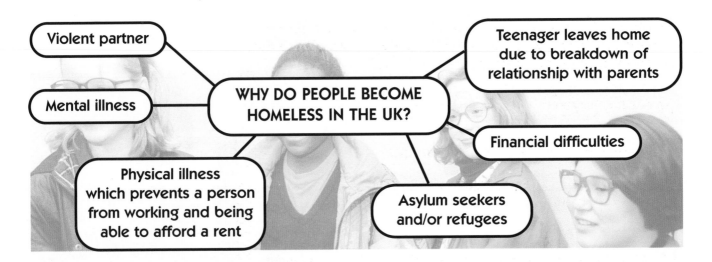

- Violent partner
- Mental illness
- Physical illness which prevents a person from working and being able to afford a rent

WHY DO PEOPLE BECOME HOMELESS IN THE UK?

- Teenager leaves home due to breakdown of relationship with parents
- Financial difficulties
- Asylum seekers and/or refugees

KEY TASKS

Talk about the effects that homelessness may have on a person. Think about the physical, intellectual, emotional and social needs of the person.

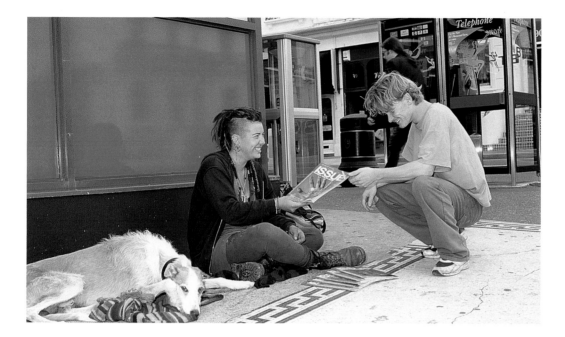

KEY TASKS

The Big Issue and the Salvation Army are two organisations that help to support people who are homeless. Find out about the organisations and write brief notes on each of them.

www.bigissue.com
www.salvationarmy.org

━━ Memory Jogger ━━

1 How can you promote equality of opportunity when working with children? Give two examples.
2 Describe what is meant by poverty.
3 Why do people become homeless? Give three reasons.

Drug abuse

For teenagers the most dangerous thing about alcohol is what happens when they are drunk. Every year over 1000 people under the age of 16 end up in hospital after drinking too much. People are more likely to get into fights after drinking and have unsafe sex. Alcohol is involved in 30% of road accidents, which are the biggest cause of death in young people under 30.

Drinking habits of 11–16 year-olds in percentage

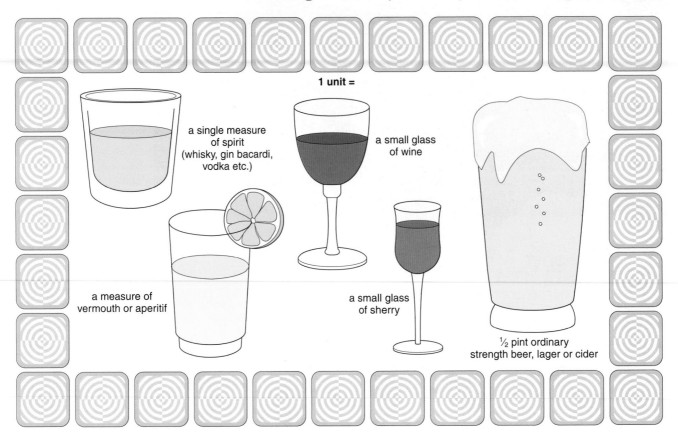

1 unit =

a single measure of spirit (whisky, gin bacardi, vodka etc.)

a small glass of wine

a measure of vermouth or aperitif

a small glass of sherry

½ pint ordinary strength beer, lager or cider

These apply to the 25ml measure used in England and Wales. A pub measure in Northern Ireland is 35ml, i.e. 1½ units. In Scotland it can either be 35ml or 25ml. Source: Health Education Board for Scotland 1999

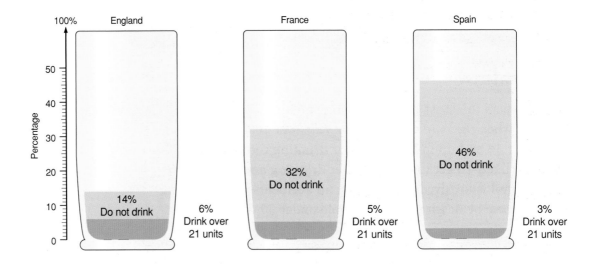

England — 14% Do not drink — 6% Drink over 21 units

France — 32% Do not drink — 5% Drink over 21 units

Spain — 46% Do not drink — 3% Drink over 21 units

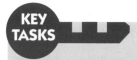

KEY TASKS

Carry out a survey to find out the drinking habits of a group of people.

① Design a simple questionnaire. The table below is an example of what you might do.

1 Do you drink alcohol?		Yes		No	
2 What is your favourite drink?	Beer	Wine	Spirits	Others
3 When do you drink most?	Mon–Thurs	Friday	Sat	Sun
4 How much do you drink in an evening?	1 unit	2 units	3 units	More

② When you have gathered the information you need, present your information in different ways, e.g. a bar chart.

Remember to include:
* a title on each chart that you draw
* titles on the X and Y axis
* a key if you have used different colours or symbols.

③ Write a short paragraph to describe what your results show.

Smoking

Nearly 40% of all adults in Britain smoke and almost all of them are aware that smoking can lead to ill health.

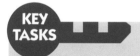

KEY TASKS

If you smoke complete the questionnaire below yourself. If you do not smoke ask someone who does.

If you smoke, why do you do it?	Yes	No
Holding a cigarette is part of the pleasure.		
It helps relieve stress and tension.		
It makes you feel good.		
You enjoy it and find it relaxing.		
You do it without thinking.		
It's important to do what your friends do.		

'Smoking in front of the children is ...'

'The Government should ... tax on cigarettes.'

'I ... when people are smoking next to me.'

'If someone smokes when I am having my hair cut I ...'

How would you complete the statements above? Discuss your opinions about smoking in a small group.

2. PREPARING FOR WORK

Before you begin to look for work in child care it is important to find out what skills and qualities you already have.

Fill in the checklist below. Be honest. You may find that you leave some boxes empty. This does not mean that you are not suitable to work with young children. It does mean that you need to gain more experience, learn new skills and learn from the course that you are studying.

Children

- [ ] Enjoy being with children.
- [ ] Willing to do the unpleasant tasks (e.g. cleaning a child who has been sick).
- [ ] Able to talk easily to children of different ages and abilities.
- [ ] Able to suggest ideas of what to do with the children (e.g. painting activities, different types of books to read to children).
- [ ] Aware of everything that is going on around you.

People

- [ ] Able to get on with people from different cultures and backgrounds.
- [ ] Able to listen to others and take advice.
- [ ] Able to work with parents and other child care workers.
- [ ] Be part of a team.
- [ ] Be sensitive to other people's feelings.
- [ ] Able to cope with 'difficult' people.
- [ ] Speak clearly to others.

Personal qualities

- [ ] Patient, lots of energy and stamina.
- [ ] Willing to learn.
- [ ] Able to learn from your mistakes.
- [ ] Able to take responsibility for your own actions.
- [ ] Stay calm in a crisis.
- [ ] Able to follow instructions.
- [ ] Maintain a high standard of personal appearance, time keeping and commitment

Once you have decided that you are interested in working with young children you will need to find out:

✴ what age of children you want to work with
✴ what type of work you want to do, e.g. in a family home or working with other adults
✴ if you need qualifications for the job you want to do
✴ what qualifications you need
✴ what experience you need, if any
✴ what age you need to be before you start working with children.

Jobs in child care

There is a wide range of jobs in child care and it is important that you find out as much as you can about each job before you decide to apply for a specific job.

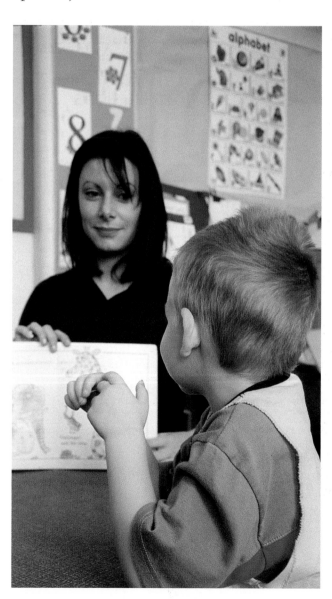

FOR THESE JOBS
YOU WILL NEED
TO HAVE OR BE
WORKING
TOWARDS A LEVEL
2 QUALIFICATION

Nursery assistant
Parent/toddler
group assistant
Nursery supervisor
Babysitter/au pair

Pre-school assistant
Mother's help
Crèche assistant
Playgroup assistant

Assistant play
worker
Play worker
Holiday scheme
play worker
Adventure play
worker

FOR THESE JOBS
YOU WILL NEED
TO HAVE A LEVEL
3 QUALIFICATION

Nursery supervisor
Pre-school leader

Crèche leader
Playgroup leader
Toy library leader
Special educational
needs supporter
Nursery Nurse
Nanny
Childminder
Senior play worker/
co-ordinator

FOR THESE JOBS YOU WILL NEED TO HAVE A LEVEL 4 QUALIFICATION

| Manager | Development officer | Advanced Practitioner |

| Play work manager | Play work development officer |

Where to find more information about jobs in child care

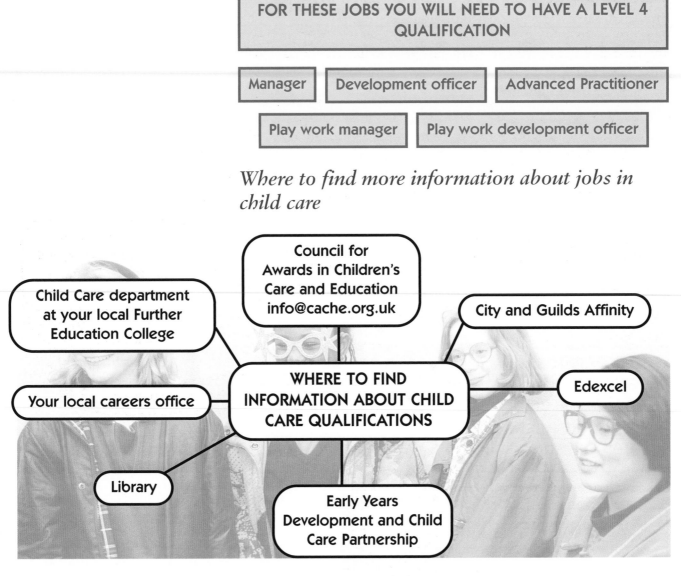

Child Care department at your local Further Education College

Council for Awards in Children's Care and Education info@cache.org.uk

City and Guilds Affinity

Your local careers office

WHERE TO FIND INFORMATION ABOUT CHILD CARE QUALIFICATIONS

Edexcel

Library

Early Years Development and Child Care Partnership

Child care qualifications

There are three different levels of child care qualifications:

* Level 2 qualifications are for people who are working under supervision in a child care setting.
* Level 3 qualifications are for people who can work on their own or are supervising other people in the child care setting.
* Level 4 qualifications are for people who are in management positions or are experienced child care workers.

Experience of working with children

When you go for an interview for a child care course or for a job, you are usually asked 'What experience do you have working with young children?'

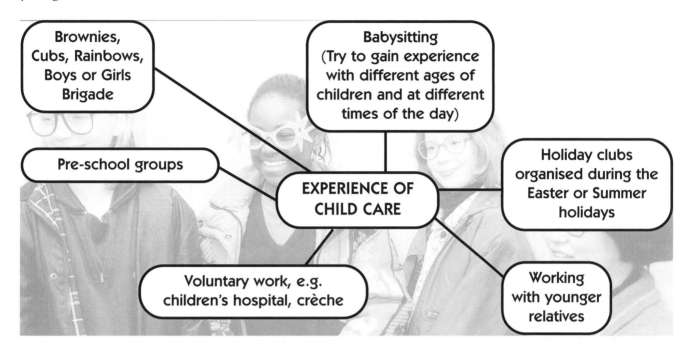

Brownies, Cubs, Rainbows, Boys or Girls Brigade

Babysitting (Try to gain experience with different ages of children and at different times of the day)

Pre-school groups

EXPERIENCE OF CHILD CARE

Holiday clubs organised during the Easter or Summer holidays

Voluntary work, e.g. children's hospital, crèche

Working with younger relatives

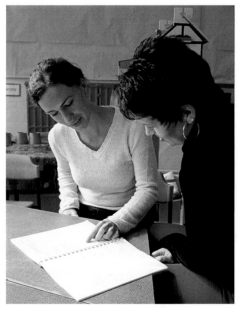

How old do you need to be to work with young children?

The Care Standards Act 2000 recommends that child care workers should be 18 years and over before they begin to work with young children. Younger people will have to work under supervision.

If you want to work towards a child care qualification at Level 2

Level 3

Level 3 Job Roles

CACHE awards can be used in a variety of environments including daycare and classroom settings. Level 3 qualifications are suitable for workers who will be working unsupervised in the following job roles:

Nursery Officer in Charge
Residential Childcare worker
Family Centre Manager
Family Careworker
Nursery Nurse
Pre-school leader
Creche leader
Childminder
Senior playworker/co-ordinator
Special educational needs supporter
Toy Library Leader

CACHE level 3 Diploma in Child Care and Education *

CACHE level 3 Certificate of Professional Development in Work with Children and Young People *

CACHE level 3 Certificate in Childminding Practice *

CACHE level 3 Diploma in Pre-school Practice

CACHE level 3 Diploma in Early Years Care and Education (Welsh Medium)

NVQ level 3 in Early Years Care and Education

NVQ level 3 in Caring for Children and Young People

NVQ level 3 in Playwork

CACHE ADCE

This award is a professional development award aimed at early years' works with several years' experience that wish to update their knowledge. It supplies the underpinning knowledge needed for NVQ level 4 and carries 120 CAT points which is equivalent to the first year of an undergraduate course

Level 4

NVQ in Early Years Care and Education level 4

This award provides a challenging opportunity to obtain a higher level of professional skills. It is suitable for people working at senior level with children or children and their families.

Qualifications featured in this leaflet are on the National Childcare Qualifications Framework
* see reverse for full details

Level 2

Level 2 Job Roles

Family Support worker in a Family Centre
Parent/Toddler Group assistant
Homestart worker
Nursery assistant
Pre-school assistant
Creche assistant
Toy Library worker
Holiday Playscheme worker
Playgroup assistant

CACHE level 2 Certificate in Child Care and Education

CACHE level 2 Certificate in Pre-school Practice

CACHE level 2 Certificate in Playwork

NVQ level 2 in Early Years Care and Education

NVQ level 2 in Playwork

These Level 2 qualifications are suitable for workers who will be working under supervision in the above job roles.

Level 1

CACHE Foundation Award in Caring for Children

Although this award is **not** a licence to practice it's used as a taster for those who are thinking of a career in Childcare (usually offered in schools and colleges of further education). It has proved useful for returnees to the workplace and in settings that are working towards, or have obtained 'Investors in People'.

Entry Level

NAMCW will be merging with CACHE this year and CACHE now offers their Entry Level Award focusing on parent craft and citizenship for young people in prisons, mother and baby units, young people in need, young parents with problems with parent craft and young people interested in parent craft in schools.

or above you must be at least 16 years of age before you start the course.

What is the law regarding babysitting?

There is no law in England or Wales to prevent anyone of any age babysitting, BUT a person under the age of 16 cannot be charged with neglect or ill-treatment of a child left in their care. Parents remain responsible and can be charged themselves if their child is harmed in any way.

In Scotland the minimum legal age for a babysitter is 16 years old, BUT even some 16 year-olds may not be mature enough to be responsible for the care of children.

Finding the right job

There are many different types of jobs in child care.

Day nurseries
They usually care for pre-school children while their parents are at work. Some day nurseries are open for 12 hours each day

Child minders
A child minder looks after children in their own home. They must be registered with Social Services and have done training.

Pre-school groups
These groups are usually held in the morning or afternoon for children before they start school. Parents pay a small fee.

JOBS IN CHILD CARE

Nannies
A nanny is employed by the parent to care for their children in the child's home. The nanny may live in the family home. The nanny will be expected to clean, cook and play with the children.

Breakfast clubs, after school clubs and holiday care
These clubs are open to children aged between 5 and 15 before and after school and during the holidays. They are run by play workers and nursery nurses.

Before you begin to apply for jobs you need to decide what type of work you are interested in.

There are a variety of different ways of finding jobs in child care.
* Local newspaper
* Job centre
* Magazines, e.g. Nursery World, The Lady
* Web site, e.g.
  www.nanny-jobs.co.uk
  www.thenannybureau.com
  www.nannies-unimited.co.uk

KEY TASKS

Use the search engine www.google.com Enter the words 'nanny jobs uk' and look at different job sites for more detailed information.

The job advertisement should tell you:

* the job title
* the qualifications and experience that are needed
* salary
* where you will be working e.g. in the child's home, at a nursery
* a brief description of the job
* how and where to apply, including a closing date.

KEY TASKS

① What are the advantages and disadvantages of the job?

② What does the job advertisement not tell you?

③ Make a list of the questions you would like to ask when you go for the interview.

Mother's help

(live out au pair) needed to help care for a five month old baby girl.

Full time Mon–Fri
9am to 5pm
£160 per week
(according to experience).
Immediate start.
phone: 0123 456789

LIVE IN MOTHER'S HELP NEEDED ASAP

Domestic duties and help with girl 3 and baby twin boys.

Non smoker, baby experience, references and reasonable English.

Double room in nice house.

Minimum 37 hours Mon–Fri plus babysitting.

£150 per week.

Write to Mr Smith explaining why you think you would be suitable for the job.

① What is the hourly rate of pay? Is it above the minimum wage?

② Make a list of the questions you would want to ask Mr Smith if you were invited for an interview.

How many children are you going to work with and what are their ages? Be realistic, do you have enough experience to manage.

Do you live in or out?

Are there any extras e.g. baby sitting, domestic duties? Do you get paid more for doing these jobs?

READ THE JOB ADVERT CAREFULLY

Smoking or non smoking. Many parents will not employ child carers if they smoke.

What is the hourly rate? The weekly rate may sound good but when you work out the hourly rate it may be very small. Remember working with young children is hard work.

How many hours a day are you going to work?

Job descriptions

A job description should explain what the job is about and what you would be expected to do.

Did you know?

Many parents will not employ child carers who smoke.

WONDERLAND PRE-SCHOOL PLAY ASSISTANT

Reports to: Play Leader

The assistant will support the play leader in providing a safe and stimulating environment for the children.

In order to achieve this, the assistant will:

* Help prepare and set out the playroom before the children arrive and tidy up after the children have left
* Help to provide and take part in activities for the children
* Take part in special events and outings
* Listen and talk with the children
* Attend team meetings
* Tell the play leader if he/she has any concerns about individual children
* Maintain confidentiality

What employers expect you to do for an application

* Fill in the application form in ink or word process it.
* Make sure all spellings are correct.
* Make sure your handwriting is neat and easy to read.
* Read the application form carefully before you begin writing.
* Put the answers in the right places.
* Give as much information as you can.
* Make sure the information is relevant.
* Remember to sign the form.
* If you are not sure about the application form, contact the employer and ask.

Keeping records of what you have done

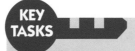

KEY TASKS

Make a list of everything you have achieved or done over the last five years.

You could include:

* Certificates you may have gained, e.g. Duke of Edinburgh Award, Girl Guide or Venture Scout badges
* Certificates from music or drama festivals
* Cycling proficiency certificate or driving test
* Certificates you may have gained for sport, e.g. swimming, athletics
* Certificates of attendance from any course you have been on
* Part-time work
* Voluntary work, e.g. Brownies, cubs, after school clubs, babysitting
* Hobbies and interests, e.g. sport, reading
* Certificates you may have gained at school
* References you may have received, e.g. from your school teacher, work experience tutor, employer.

Did you find it easy trying to remember everything you have done?

If you do not make a note of your achievements as they happen you may forget some and this could be important when you apply for a college course or a job.

A National Record of Achievement (ROA) is one way of keeping a record of what you have achieved. If you do not have a ROA you can compile your own. All you need is a file to keep your certificates and references in.

Writing a Curriculum Vitae

A Curriculum Vitae (CV) tells your employer about your education and employment experience.

Always word process your CV if possible and only use two sides of A4 paper. However do not make the font so small that no one can read it.

CVs are written in different ways and there are software packages available to help you. The important thing to remember is that the information should be easy to find, clear and accurate. There is an example of a CV on page 38.

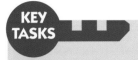

KEY TASKS

Write your own CV and word process it. Save your work on a disc so that you can update it when you have completed your child care course.

WRITING A LETTER OF APPLICATION

Sometimes you will be asked to write a letter of application instead of, or as well as, a CV. This will take time to write so do not leave it to the last minute.

✸ Look at the closing date for the application. You will need to post your letter at least two days before to be sure that it arrives on time. If possible hand deliver it.

✸ Use good quality A4 paper.

✸ Make a rough copy of the letter. Word process it if possible. Always check your final work for any spelling errors, missing words and accuracy. It can be useful to ask someone else to read it.

✸ Make a photocopy of your letter or save it on disc. You can then read it again before you go for your interview.

✸ When you write the letter use the job description to help you.

✸ Use a matching envelope.

A letter of application has been written for the position of Play Assistant at the Wonderland Pre-school. It can be found on page 39. The job description is shown on page 40.

Curriculum Vitae

Name:	Ann Isdale	*Date of Birth:*	30.10.1985
Address:	38 Ashley Terrace New Town NT12 34RE	*Telephone No:*	01234 567890
National Insurance No:	KV1234 5678	*Nationality:*	Scottish
		Marital status:	Single

Education

September 1996 – Present	Muir High School, New Town, NT12 34RE
Course September 1999 – Present	CACHE Foundation Award in Caring for Young Children

Work Experience

June 2000	Tiny Tots Day Nursery (Age 2/4 yrs) 15 days

Qualifications

Subject	Board	Date	Grade
English	NEB	July 2000	E
ICT	NEB	July 2000	E

Employment

June 1999 – present	J R Brown Stationery Shop Saturday only Serve customers, operate cash machine

Interests and hobbies

Help with Rainbows each week
Enjoy swimming
Play the piano

Referees

Ms I Gills Personal Tutor Muir High School New Town NT12 34RE	Mr D Green Work experience supervisor Tiny Tots Day Nursery New Town NT15 2KL

Mr J Smith
Wonderland Pre-school
London
AB1 2CD

21 May 2001

Miss A Philips
12 Straight Road
Main Town
EF3 4GH

Dear Mr Smith

Re: Position of Play Assistant

I would like to apply for the position of play assistant at Wonderland Pre-School.

When I was studying on the CACHE Foundation in Caring for Young Children, I spent three weeks on work experience at a pre-school group with 3–4 year old children. I helped to prepare the activities for the children and tidied up at the end of the day.

I have also helped at my church crèche with babies from a few weeks old to two years.

When I work with the children I like to listen and talk to them. I also like to play with them. I try to give them ideas but I do not force them to do what I say.

During the summer holidays I look after my four year old cousin. We go to the park and the swimming pool each week. I have to watch Peter all the time to stop him having an accident.

When I was on my work experience I went to the team meetings. My supervisor always asked me to share ideas about new activities that I could do with the children. My supervisor used to ask me if I found some children difficult to work with. She always reminded me about confidentiality.

I also go to meetings for the church crèche. We plan the Christmas party and what we are going to do each week.

I am very interested in the play assistant's job and I have included my CV to give you extra information.

Yours sincerely

Ann Philips

This is the address of the person you want to send the letter to.

This is the date when you write the letter.

This is your address.

You can write all this information in a straight line.

This is the name of the potential employer.

You should name the job that you want to apply for and where it is.

Go through each section of the job description explaining what experience you have had.

This section is about number 1 in the job description on page 40. Try to give as much information as possible.

Although this is not the age group that you would be working with, it tells the employer that you know a little about the younger children and you are interested in working with children in your spare time.

This section is about number 2 and number 4. Show that you know what your role is in providing and taking part in activities.

This section is about number 3. This is not full time experience but again it shows that you are interested in working with children in your spare time.

This section is about number 5, 6 and 7.

When you have given as much information as you can you need to finish the letter. Include your CV if you can. It will give the employer more information about yourself.

If you know the person's name you finish your letter with 'Yours sincerely'. If you do not know the person's name your finish your letter with 'Yours faithfully'.

It is useful to print your name and then sign it above.

Wonderland Pre-school Job Description

Play Assistant

Reports to: Play Leader

The assistant will support the play leader in providing a safe and stimulating environment for the children.

In order to achieve this, the assistant will:

What experience do you have of setting out playrooms etc? Think back to your work experience.

1. Help prepare and set out the playroom before the children arrive and tidy up after the children have left

What activities have you provided for children of this age group? Remember all the experience you have had during work experience and any voluntary work you have done with children e.g. babysitting.

2. Help to provide and take part in activities for the children

Have you taken children on outings or organised special events e.g. birthdays?

3. Take part in special events and outings

What experience have you had of listening and talking with children?

4. Listen and talk with the children

You may not have had experience of child care team meetings but have you had team meetings in your part time work?

5. Attend team meetings

What experience have you had of sharing information with other adults e.g. parent of the child you are babysitting for?

6. Tell the play leader if he/she has any concerns about individual children

What experience have you had on maintaining confidentiality?

7. Maintain confidentiality

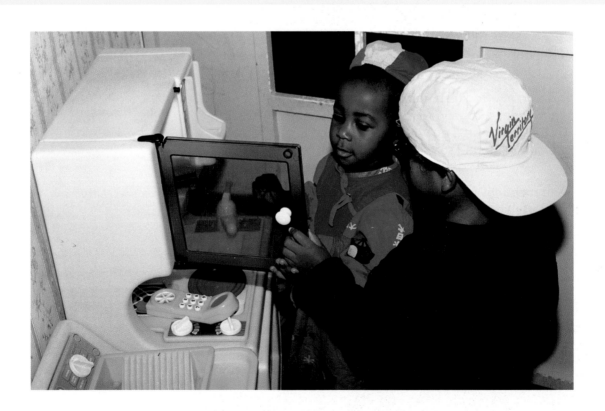

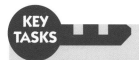

Write a letter of application for the Wonderland Pre-School position. It will take time and it will not be easy, but the notes on page 39 should help you.

Preparing for an interview

Be smart and on time

Always make an effort when you go for an interview. The employer wants to talk to someone who is clean, tidy and smartly dressed. Do not wear your old jeans and T-shirt.

KEY TASKS

Imagine you are the employer at Wonderland Pre-school. Now look at the pictures below of possible applicants. Who would you offer the job of play assistant to? Give reasons for your answer.

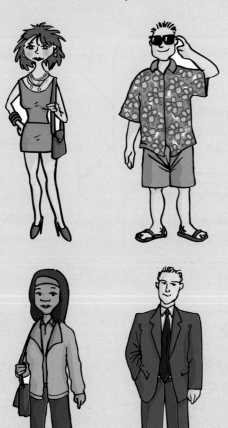

Know where you are going

Make sure you know where you are going and give yourself plenty of time to get there. It can be useful to go a few days before the interview to make sure you do not get lost.

Be prepared

When you go for an interview you will be asked different types of questions. Some will be about yourself, what experience you have and what interests and hobbies you have. Other questions will test your knowledge of how to care for young children.

Take your National Record of Achievement with you and any other reports that may be useful, e.g. you may take some of your college work with you.

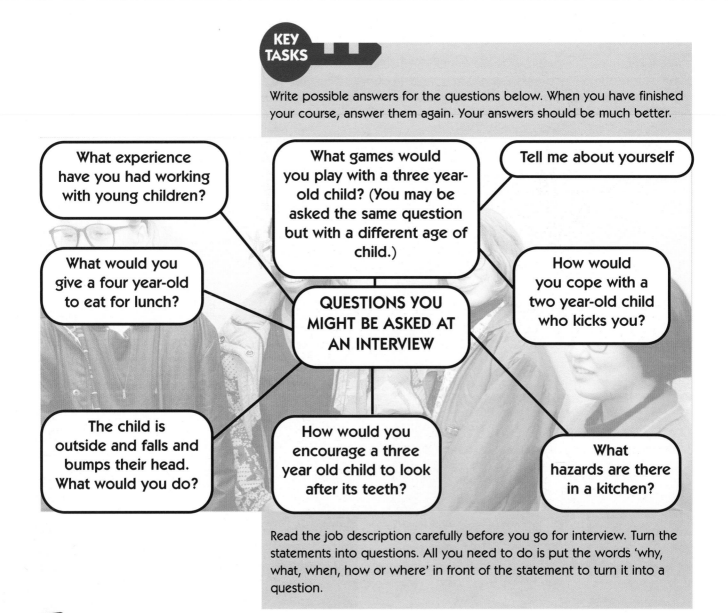

KEY TASKS

Write possible answers for the questions below. When you have finished your course, answer them again. Your answers should be much better.

What experience have you had working with young children?

What games would you play with a three year-old child? (You may be asked the same question but with a different age of child.)

Tell me about yourself

What would you give a four year-old to eat for lunch?

QUESTIONS YOU MIGHT BE ASKED AT AN INTERVIEW

How would you cope with a two year-old child who kicks you?

The child is outside and falls and bumps their head. What would you do?

How would you encourage a three year old child to look after its teeth?

What hazards are there in a kitchen?

Read the job description carefully before you go for interview. Turn the statements into questions. All you need to do is put the words 'why, what, when, how or where' in front of the statement to turn it into a question.

Be calm

Be as calm and relaxed as possible. You will be nervous but if you are well prepared you will do your best. Do not be too disappointed if you do not get the job. It is good experience and you will have learned a great deal from it. Use the experience the next time and you may well be successful.

KEY TASKS

Look at the job description below. The statements have been turned into questions. Can you answer them?

Job Description

Post Parent help

Job summary To help the parent look after 3 year old twins from 8am until 6pm, 5 days a week.

Main duties	Possible questions
1 Help the parent look after the children	1 How can I help the parent look after the children?
2 Help to carry out general duties e.g. bathing the children, preparing meals for the family, washing and ironing the family's clothes	2 How will I bath the children? How will I prepare meals for the family making sure that it is safe and hygienic?
3 Play with the children	3 What will I play with the children? Remember to look at the ages of the children.
4 Clean and tidy up the children's room and any areas the children use.	4 How will I make sure that the children's areas are clean and tidy?
5 Maintain a safe environment for the children	5 How will I make sure that the environment is safe?
6 Ensure confidentiality at all times	6 What will I do to ensure confidentiality?
7 Keep your own room clean and tidy	7 Why is it important to keep my own room clean and tidy?

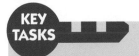

KEY TASKS

Use the job description for the Wonderland Pre-school and make the statements into questions. Try to answer each question. (You could use this task at the end of your course to help you to revise for your short answer paper.)

3. WORKING EFFECTIVELY WITH OTHERS

Organising your time

How good are you at organising your time?

	YES	NO	SOMETIMES
1 Do you get to classes on time?			
2 If you have agreed to meet your friend in town, do you get there first?			
3 Are you always rushing at the last minute to get your course work finished?			
4 Do you have time to relax without feeling guilty that you should be doing something else?			
5 Do you manage to do everything you want to in a week?			

Going to classes

Sleeping and eating

Going to work experience

Studying for the examination

Going out with your friends

Working on portfolio tasks

Travelling to and from school/college

Having time for yourself, e.g. listening to music

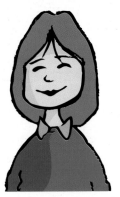

When you are working on a course, you will have a lot to do in a very short period of time.

KEY TASKS

* Make a list of all the things that you have to do over the next week.

* Use a highlighting pen to show which tasks are the most important.

* Use a different colour of pen to highlight the tasks that can wait.

* How long will you need to spend on each task?

* Put the most tasks that must be done on a notice board in your room or make a note of them in your diary.

* Tick them off when you have done each task.

Sometimes it is useful to draw a plan for the week and use different colours of pen to show the most important tasks.

Working in a team

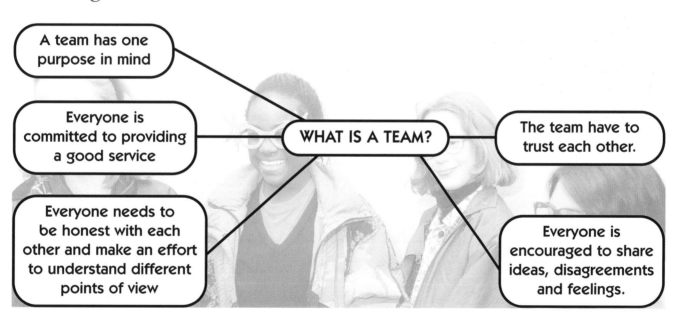

A team has one purpose in mind

Everyone is committed to providing a good service

Everyone needs to be honest with each other and make an effort to understand different points of view

WHAT IS A TEAM?

The team have to trust each other.

Everyone is encouraged to share ideas, disagreements and feelings.

When you work as a member of a team you will be able to:

* learn from others who have more experience than you
* see things from other people's points of view
* share ideas
* ask and answer questions, which will help you to understand the job better
* learn to accept criticism
* get help and support when faced with challenges or difficult tasks.

Being part of a team

When you are working as part of a team you will be expected to:

✳ listen to other members of the team
✳ be sensitive to the feelings of other team members
✳ encourage others in the team because they will encourage you.

How good are you at the job?

Whatever job or task you are doing, it is always important to ask yourself if you are doing the best job that you can. It is important to be as honest as you can.

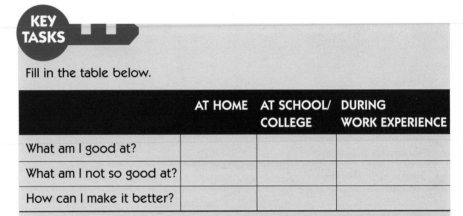

KEY TASKS

Fill in the table below.

	AT HOME	AT SCHOOL/ COLLEGE	DURING WORK EXPERIENCE
What am I good at?			
What am I not so good at?			
How can I make it better?			

Ask a friend to tell you what they think you are good at and what you are not so good at?

4. WORKING EFFECTIVELY IN A CHILD CARE SETTING

What is expected of you?

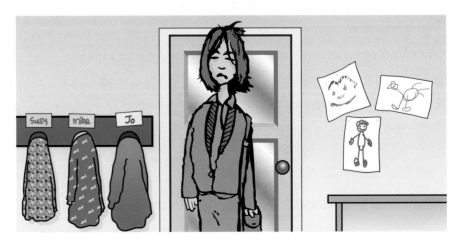

To work with young children you need to:

✳ Enjoy the work. A person who arrives at work each day feeling fed up, grumpy and not interested will not be able to do a good job.

✳ Be interested in helping children learn

✳ Be able to talk to young children and build a good relationship with them

✳ Be patient, have lots of energy and stamina

✳ Be able to work with other adults

✳ Be prepared to do anything, e.g. changing nappies, cleaning equipment, clean out the animals, read stories …

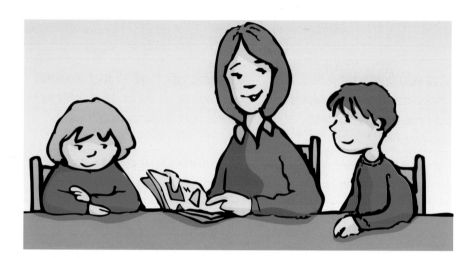

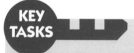
KEY TASKS

On your first day on work experience, find out:

THINGS TO FIND OUT
① Where the fire exits are
② What you do when the fire alarm sounds
③ What you do if a child injures itself
④ Where the protective gloves are kept in the work setting
⑤ Who you report accidents to
⑥ Who you talk to if a child is unwell
⑦ What you do if you hear a child using racist language or is bullying another child

PRACTICAL HINTS FOR WORK EXPERIENCE

BE ON TIME AND RELIABLE	TALK TO THE OTHER MEMBERS OF THE TEAM	BE AWARE OF SAFETY
Find out what hours you are expected to work.	Ask if you do not understand what you should be doing. You will learn more by doing this.	You need 'eyes in the back of your head' to work with young children.
Check the times of the buses, trains, etc to make sure that you are not late. Remember the children will be there on time.	Tell your supervisor what you have learned about the children.	You must be aware of their safety at all times.
Remember that your working hours does not include changing into a uniform, having a drink before you start etc.	Ask your supervisor to explain how you are getting on in the work setting. Do not leave it until the last day of your placement.	Never become so involved with a group of children that you are not aware of what other children are doing around in different areas of the work setting.
If you are ill, let your supervisor know as soon as possible. They will be expecting you.	Tell your supervisor if your are not happy. He/she may be able to help you.	Sit on the child sized seats or stand in a position that lets you see as much of the play area as possible.
If you are asked to prepare an activity or bring in objects from home, do not let the children or the team members down.	Watch how the other members of staff work with the children. Remember they have a lot of experience and you can learn a lot from them.	

KEY TASKS

Talk to other students who have completed work experience in the child care setting. What did they enjoy? What did they find difficult? What advice would they give you for your first day?

Introduction to students and visiting helpers

We would like to welcome you to the nursery. The staff here works very much as a team and we will expect you to join in with us as one of that team.

Please feel able to ask either of us about any problems or questions you have at any time. We will do the same – if we are not happy about any aspect of your work, we will speak to you about it, not with a view to criticising, but with the intention of helping you to get the best from your time with us.

Members of staff discuss children, but always with a view to the child's needs and to finding ways of taking the child on to the next stage of their development. Hopefully it is never done for reasons of 'gossip'. We must always respect the individual and we expect you to treat any information you hear as confidential, as we do ourselves.

How to Start

It is best to start by watching what is happening. Observe everything and everybody in the nursery i.e. the equipment, the layout of the room and its surroundings. What are the routines? How is snack time, gym, TV etc organised? When do the children wear aprons? When do they have their names written and how? How many children are allowed at each of the activities etc.

Observe the children

Get down to their level and watch how they talk and play with each other. Who are the dominant children? Who are the quiet withdrawn ones? What are their names? Which activities are the most popular and why?

Observe the staff

How do they speak to the children? How do they give them instructions? How do they allocate tasks?

In other words, find out everything you can in your first few days. In this way you will quickly become a member of the team.

Chirnside Nursery Class

KEY TASKS

Read the leaflet above and answer the questions.

1. Why will the staff talk to you if they are not happy about the work you are doing?
2. Why does the staff discuss children in the nursery?
3. Why is it important not to talk about children outside the nursery?
4. Why is it important to observe the children and the staff in your first few days at the nursery?
5. Give **three** examples of what you should observe.

Punctuality	You are expected to arrive at the nursery in good time, to help the other team members prepare the activities for the day.
Absence	You must let the nursery know as soon as possible.
Dress	You should be clean, neat and tidy and wear clothes, which are suitable for the activities that are being prepared for the day. You must wear the nursery apron when doing craft activities or baking with the children.
Confidentiality	You will hear confidential information about the children. On no account must this information be repeated or discussed with others.
Staff expectations	You will use you common sense and initiative when working with the children. You will help with tasks such as clearing up, helping children, washing equipment etc. without being asked.
	You will carry out all staff instructions. Everyone in the nursery is involved in all tasks including the unpleasant ones.
	You must talk to the teacher or nursery nurse about any activities that you want to do with the children. The activities must fit in with what the other staff are doing.
Candidate handbook	You must bring your candidate handbook to the nursery every day to let the teacher and nursery nurse know what you should be completing for school/college.
Managing children's behaviour	This is the teacher and nursery nurse's responsibility. Ask for help.
	Never smack or use other forms of corporal punishment.
Flexibility	Be prepared to try anything.
Attitudes to children	Be positive and enjoy being with them.
	Children quickly sense when adults are bored, tired etc.
	Speak clearly using appropriate words and grammar.
	Never speak down to a child.
	Never swear in front of the child.
	Listen to what the children are saying.
	Respond to what the children are doing.
	Do not be tempted to be too helpful. The nursery is trying to encourage the children to be independent.
	Be realistic about what the children can do.
Your daily routine	Setting out and preparing activities/materials
	Joining in structured activities e.g. baking, craft, story telling

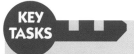

KEY TASKS

Read the leaflet on page 50 and answer these questions.

① Why is it important to arrive in good time at the nursery?

② What do you do if you are not feeling well and cannot go to the nursery?

③ What do you do if a child is being very difficult with you?

④ What must you never do if a child is not doing what he/she is being asked to do?

⑤ What attitudes should you have towards the children? Give **four** examples.

Confidentiality

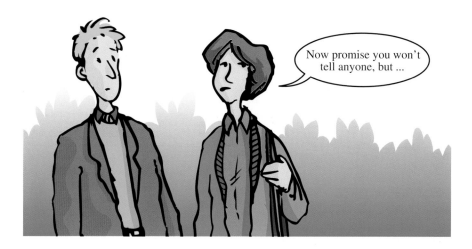

When you work with young children and their families, you may hear or read information that is confidential i.e. should not be discussed with anyone or written down. Confidentiality is the right of every child and parent whether the information is spoken, written down or entered onto a computer.

If the information you receive is likely to put the person into danger then you should tell the person that you are going to speak to your supervisor.

It is a very serious matter if you tell anyone else about the information that you have received. You may be asked to leave your placement and you may not be able to complete your course.

TEST YOURSELF

1. What does 'being a good citizen' mean?

2. What rights do you have as a British citizen? Give two examples.

3. Name two laws that affect the rights of the child.

4. What is the minimum wage for an adult?

5. What is meant by 'equality of opportunity'?

6. Why is it important to maintain confidentiality when working with children and their families?

7. How can you prepare for a job interview? Give three examples.

8. What does discrimination mean?

9. Why is the Children Act important?

10. What effect does inequality have on a child? Give three examples.

Human Growth and Development

CHAPTER 2

* How do we grow and develop?
* What affects our growth and development?

1. HOW DO WE GROW AND DEVELOP?

There are many different stages in a person's life span. They can be
divided into five main life stages. The ages given below are
approximate because everyone grows and develops at different rates.

Infancy	0–3 years
Childhood	4–9 years
Adolescence	10–18 years
Adulthood	19–65 years
Later life	65+

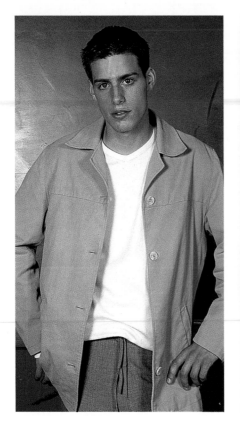
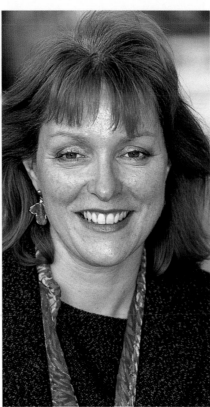
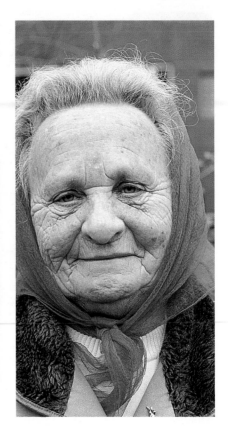

KEY TASKS

Other names are used for the main life stages. Complete the table using the words below.

Infancy			
Childhood			
Adolescence			
Adulthood			
Later life			

Baby	teenager	pensioner	pre-school
Youth	toddler	middle-aged	school-aged
Elderly	old age	puberty	

Can you think of any others?

Everyone is different

No two people are the same. We all have our own unique appearance and personality.

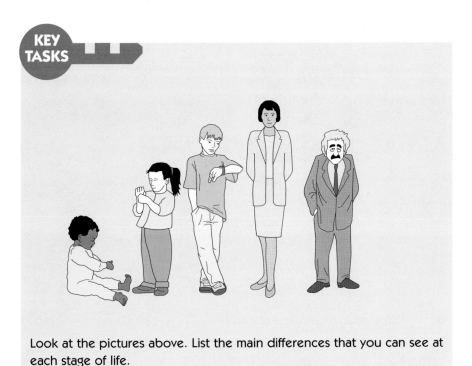

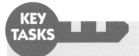

Look at the pictures above. List the main differences that you can see at each stage of life.

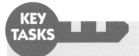

✳ Think of two different families that you know well. List all the things that you know they can do either at home, at work or in their spare time. Do not give the names of the people in the family. Your information should always be confidential.

✳ List the people that are in your family. What do they look like? What do they do? How do they spend their time?

All families are different and the people within a family are different.

What is meant by 'ages and stages'?

'Ages and stages' refers to the way we grow and develop at different times in our lives.

What does 'physical growth' mean?

Physical growth is about the changes that take place in the height, weight and length of a person.

In the first few years children develop and grow faster than at any other time in life. As children grow up they change physically, intellectually, socially and emotionally.

What does 'human development' mean?

'Development' is about the skills and capabilities of a person.

We grow and develop from birth until we reach a peak during adulthood. Then we begin to slow down until we die in old age.

AREAS OF DEVELOPMENT

Human development is usually divided up into five different areas.

① Physical development ② Intellectual development

③ Language development ④ Emotional development

⑤ Social development

Physical development is about:

✳ The structure of the body i.e. the nervous system (brain and nerves), respiratory system (nose, air passages, lungs), reproductive system (ovaries, uterus)
✳ How each aspect of the body relates to each other
✳ How the body grows and develops
✳ The factors which affect the physical development of the body

> **Did you know?**
>
> Each person's development will follow a similar pattern but it will take place at different rates.

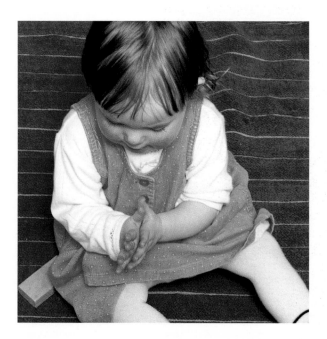
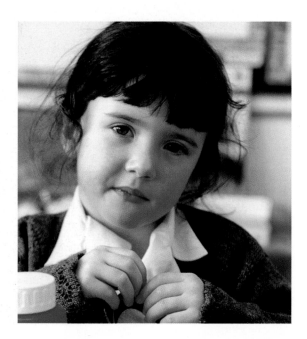

Intellectual development is about:

* Solving problems
* Remembering (memory)
* Concentration
* Imagination and creativity
* Working things out (reasoning)

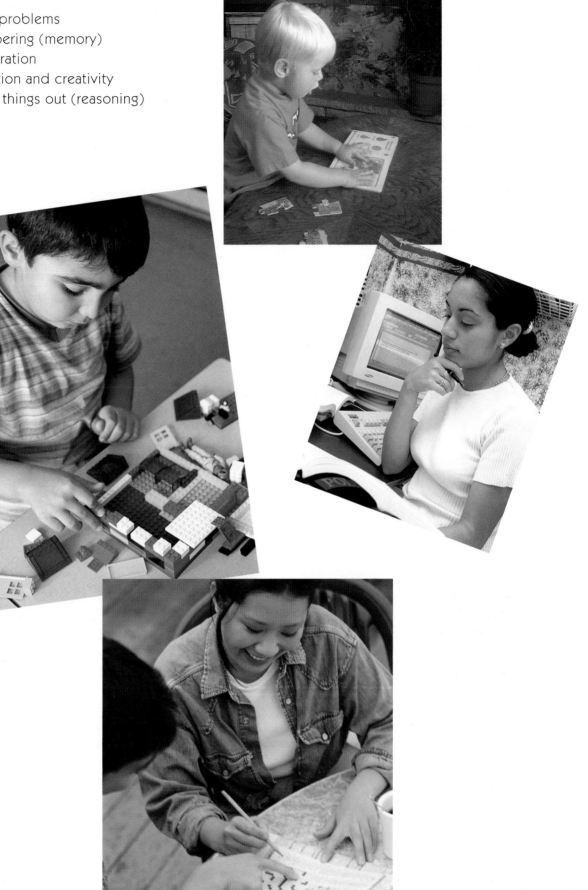

Language development is about:

* Reading
* Writing
* Listening
* Talking

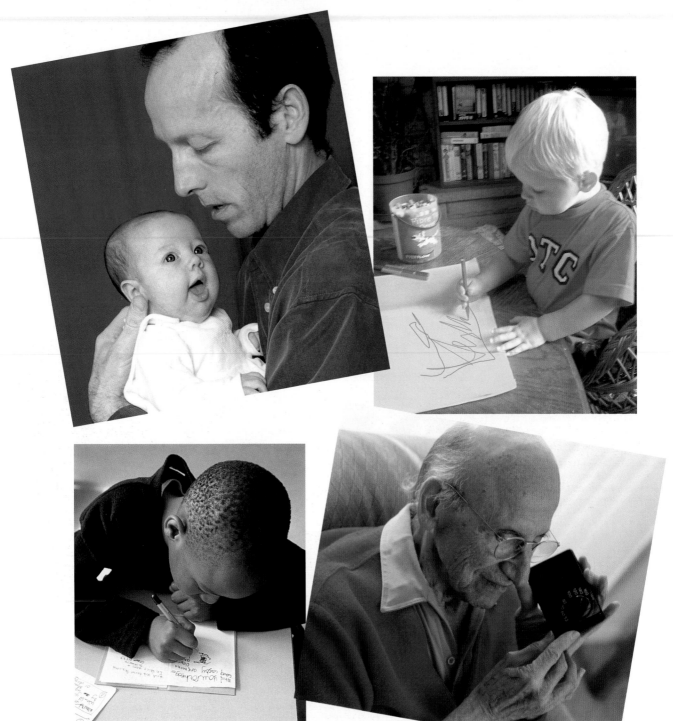

Emotional development is about:

* Making sense of your feelings
* Developing feelings towards other people
* Building up your self image
* Becoming aware of your own identity

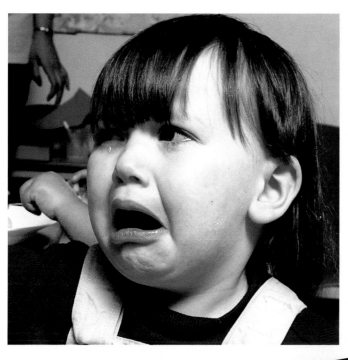

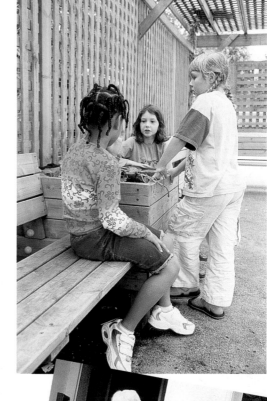

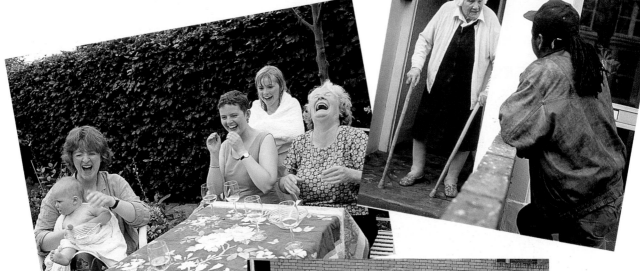

Social development is about:

* Getting on with other people
* Making friends
* Developing social skills, e.g. knowing how to behave in different situations
* Learning how to become part of a community

Physical development

Develop fine manipulative skills

Develop control over their body

Develop spatial awareness

Develop gross motor skills

Develop hand and eye co-ordination

Social development

Be aware of the needs of others and their feelings

Learn from positive role models

Share with one another

Take turns

Have a sense of responsibility

Be indepedent

Play and work with people of all ages

Emotional development

Understanding the difference between right and wrong

Understand and cope with difficult experiences, e.g. starting a new nursery

Coping with fears and anxieties, e.g. going into hospital

Build up confidence

Enjoy a sense of achievement

Learn in a secure environment

Learn how to show feelings

Make choices

Encourage self esteem

Human Development

Intellectual development

Develop thought processes	Develop concentration skills
Develop reasoning skills	Improve memory
Use the senses in order to understand the world around us	Develop creativity and imagination
Develop mathematical and scientific skills	

Language development

Learn new vocabulary	Talk in simple and complex sentences
Develop listening skills	Ask and answer questions
Read from a variety of different resources	Listen to others
Develop communication skills	Develop writing skills

Memory Jogger

What areas of development do the following statements refer to? You may find that there is more than one answer.

1. A two year-old child is having a temper tantrum in the supermarket.
2. Mary is five years-old and loves reading books.
3. Ahmid and Peter are playing together at the sand tray.
4. Kenneth enjoys playing at the wood table. He can bang the nails in hard until they almost disappear.
5. A four-year-old child is threading beads to make a necklace.
6. An adult is doing a crossword.
7. Teenagers are dancing at the local disco.
8. Moira is forty years of age and she is outside cutting the grass in her garden.
9. Susan is going into hospital for a small operation. She has never been before and is quite scared.
10. Shakila loves to play with her friends in the adventure playground.

Try making up some statements yourself and test your friends on them. Make sure you know the answers.

PHYSICAL DEVELOPMENT

There are **two** main areas of physical development that are developed:

1. Gross motor skills, i.e. large movements like running, skipping, hopping. The large muscles in the body are used.

2. Fine manipulative skills, i.e. small precise movement of the hands like writing, sewing or picking up small objects.

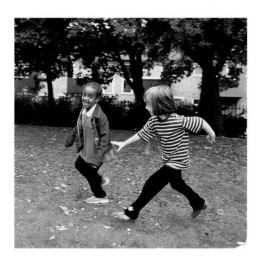
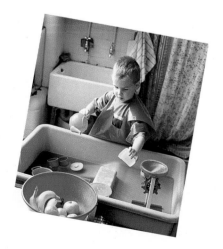

We often need to use more than one skill at a time e.g. threading a needle involves fine motor skills and hand and eye co-ordination.

Infancy: 0–3 years

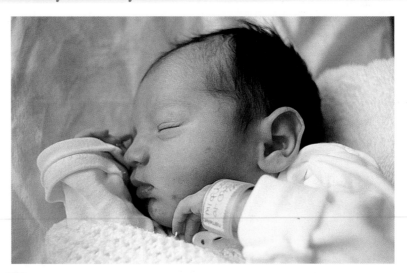

KEY TASKS

① What does a new born baby look like?

② Describe the physical appearance of the new born baby in the photograph above. You should give information about the baby's face, hair and body. You should also look at the way the baby is lying and what he/she is doing with his arms, hands and legs.

Gross motor skills

Babies

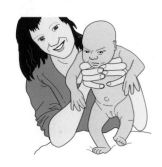

✳ When lifted the head falls backwards, if not held by the adult
✳ Turn head to light or sound
✳ Begin to take their fist to their mouths
✳ Grasp adult fingers in the hands
✳ The baby makes forward movements if held with its feet touching the ground. (walking reflex)

Three months

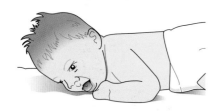

✳ Begins to have some head control
✳ Lift head and chest up
✳ Kicks

Six months

* Complete head control
* Can sit with help from an adult or the back of a chair
* Can roll from back to stomach
* Reaches out for a toy
* Uses straight arms to lift the head and chest off the ground
* Enjoys being held securely by the adult and bounced up and down

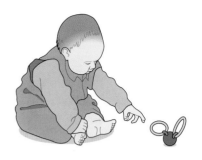

Nine months

* Pulls up into a sitting position
* Sits without help for a short time
* Holds on to furniture when standing
* Can move around the floor either by using the hands to pull and push or by rolling

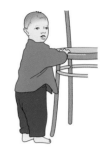

Twelve months

* Sits up without help and can turn sideways
* Stands up with help from people or by holding on to furniture
* Stands without help for a few moments
* Crawls using hands and knees or like a bear on hands and feet
* Moves by shuffling along on bottom
* Can walk with one hand held by the adult
* Walks with feet apart

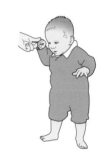

Fifteen months

* Can walk alone
* Unsteady on feet to begin with
* Able to crawl up stairs using hands and legs

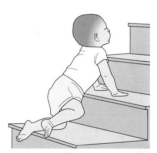

Two years

* Walks up and down stairs, two feet to one step
* Can walk on tip toe and jump

Three years

* Walks up stairs properly
* Enjoys jumping off the bottom step

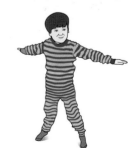

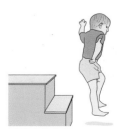

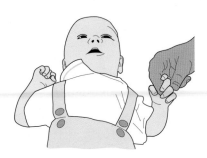

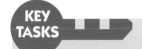

KEY TASKS

A child care student has been asked to prepare an activity for a one year old child which will help to promote her gross motor skills. The student has decided to play football with the child outside.

① Is this a good activity for the child? Give reasons for your answer.

② Suggest an activity that would be better.

Fine manipulative skills

Baby

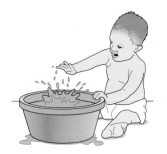

* Keeps hands tightly closed most of the time
* If anything is put into the hand, the baby will automatically grasp it tightly. This is known as the **grasp reflex** and will disappear after a few weeks

Three months

* Hands are held open for most of the time
* Grasp reflex has gone
* Holds a rattle or toy for a few moments and then drops it

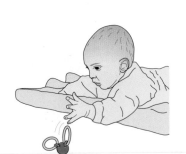

Six months

* Can grasp an object or toy without the adult putting it into the baby's hand
* Uses whole hand to hold the object
* Likes to use hands to splash water

Nine months

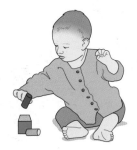

* Holds objects between the finger and thumb

Twelve months

* Holds crayon using palmer grasp
* Turns lots of pages in a book at the same time
* Drops toys deliberately and watches to see where they have fallen
* Picks up small objects using the thumb and first finger
* Uses index finger to point at interesting objects
* Uses hands to throw things

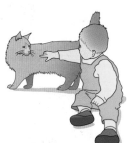

Fifteen months

* Takes cup and spoon to mouth
* Can put one brick on top of another to build a tower

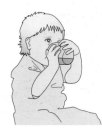

Two years

* Can put on shoes

* Begins to draw
* Turns door handles
* Enjoys building towers with at least six bricks on it

Three years

* Begins to dress themselves
* Needs help with buttons and zips

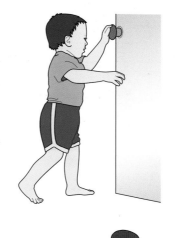
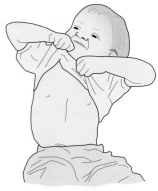

Childhood: 4–9 years

Gross motor skills

Four years

* Able to go up and down stairs using alternate feet
* Has a good sense of balance
* Can throw, catch and kick a ball
* Rides a three wheeled bicycle

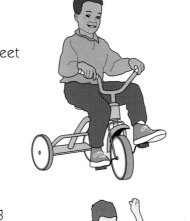
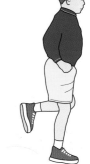

Five years

* Can skip and hop
* Runs in and out of objects or other people
* Becoming more skilled at throwing and catching different sizes of balls

Six years

* Gaining in strength and agility
* Catches, throws and kicks ball with accuracy
* Rides a two wheeled bicycle

Seven–nine years

* May be good at using roller blades
* Increased stamina
* May use one hand to catch ball

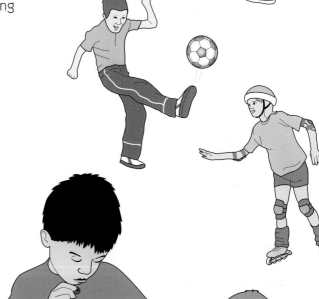

Fine manipulative skills

Four years

* Threads beads onto a string
* Holds a pencil in an adult way

Five years

* Dresses and undresses without help
* Fits smaller jigsaw pieces together
* Good control of paintbrushes and pencils

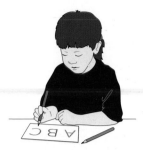

Six years

* Writes with increasing control
* Letters and numbers become smaller

Seven–nine years

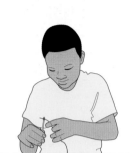

* Can thread small needle for sewing
* Greater control when writing

Adolescence: 10–18 years

* Reproductive systems do not grow very much until puberty (11–16 years) and then they grow quickly to reach adult size
* Develop a greater understanding of relationships with people of different ages
* Become independent
* Ready for work or begin employment

Physical changes of an adolescent

Several physical changes occur during the teenage years.

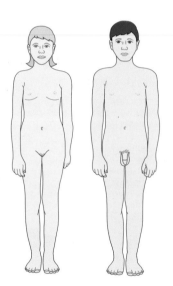

Girl
* Body hair grows
* Becomes taller and gains weight
* Breasts develop
* Periods start

Boy
* Body hair grows
* Penis and testicles develop
* Voice drops in tone or 'breaks'
* Becomes taller and gains weight

Adulthood: 19–65 years

During adulthood there are no major physical changes until women reach the menopause i.e. the end of their reproductive life. This usually happens when the woman is 45 to 55 years old, but it varies from one person to another.

* Menstruation stops and the reproductive organs shrink
* May have hot flushes and night sweats
* Osteoporosis may develop i.e. the bones become more brittle and are more likely to fracture or break

Other physical changes for men and women:

✳ Loss of hair
✳ Increased weight due to lack of exercise

Later life: 65+

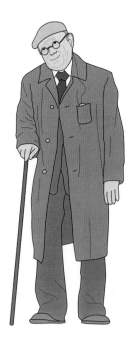

✳ Skin becomes wrinkled
✳ Bruise easily because the blood capillaries become more fragile
✳ Some loss of sight and hearing
✳ Cannot react as quickly
✳ Less steady in walking
✳ The sense of taste and smell become less effective
✳ Breathing, circulation and heart are less efficient
✳ Joints become less mobile
✳ Height decreases

Memory Jogger

Tick the appropriate age.

	0–3	4–9	10–18	19–65	65+
Becomes more skilled at throwing and catching different sized balls					
May have hot flushes and night sweats					
Pulls up into a sitting position					
Joints become less mobile					
Voice drops in tone or 'breaks'					
Rides a three wheeled bike					
May lose hair					
Skin becomes wrinkled					
Walks up stairs, one foot to one step					
Periods start					

INTELLECTUAL DEVELOPMENT

Infancy: 0–3 years

Birth to six months

✳ Use senses to find out more about their environment around them

✳ Like bright colours and interesting sounds

✳ Explores different tastes, smells and touch during feeding

✳ Begin to tell the difference between familiar sights, tastes and sounds and unfamiliar sights, tastes and sounds

✳ Understands that if an object is looked at in different ways it is still the same object

✳ Can tell the difference between simple shapes, e.g. circle, squares and triangles

Six months to twelve months

✳ Begin to understand that objects still exist even though they cannot see them

✳ Enjoy repeating actions, e.g. dropping objects and waiting until the adult picks it up

✳ Gradually understands that by dropping objects he/she has control over the adult

✳ Watch adults and try to copy them

✳ Will look for toys that have fallen from the pram or chair

✳ Can distinguish between different things and people

✳ Beginning to understand the world around them

✳ Has a short attention span, easily distracted

One to two years

✳ Increased curiosity

✳ Able to explore the environment as the child is more mobile

✳ Plays with a range of different objects

✳ Can follow simple instructions

✳ Uses an object to represent something in real life, e.g. a teddy becomes a baby

✳ Enjoys talking to themselves and copying others

✳ Beginning to show either right handedness or left handedness

✳ Can point to parts of the body and other familiar objects

✳ Can do simple jigsaws and puzzles, e.g. putting shapes into matching holes

✳ Can only concentrate on one thing at a time

Three years

✳ Begins to understand the meaning of positional words, e.g. under, over, on top of

✳ Enjoys listening to stories and joining in

✳ Knows the name of some colours, e.g. red, blue

✳ The child can move from one task to another and back again as long as there are no distractions

Childhood: 4–9 years

Four years

* Learns by watching other children and adults
* Enjoys solving problems
* Can begin to control their own concentration span. They can stop what they are doing and go back to the task without help from the adult

Five years

* Draws detailed pictures
* Enjoys solving problems
* Can listen to instructions, without stopping what they are doing and then return to the task

Seven to nine years

* Able to think in a more complex way
* Begin to understand that things are not always what they seem
* Understand what volume, weight, quantity means
* Begin to understand someone else's point of view
* Able to listen, watch and do simple things at the same time

Adolescence: 10–18 years

* Able to think in a more complex way
* Will sit formal examinations at school e.g. GCSE, GNVQ, AS and A Level
* Develops knowledge in a variety of different subjects
* Can think about things that are not actually there i.e. abstract thinking
* Questions what he/she is being told
* Develops a sense of values

Adulthood: 19–65 years

* Completed full time education
* Continuing to learn by going to short courses or taking other qualifications
* Abstract thinking
* Can think very quickly
* Good memory

Later life: 65+

* Similar to adulthood
* Cannot react as quickly

✳ Loss of memory
✳ More easily distracted

LANGUAGE DEVELOPMENT

There are four main areas of language development.

Infancy: 0–3 years

Birth to three months

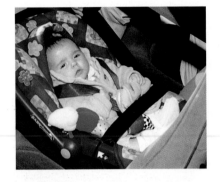

✳ Cries when hungry or wet
✳ Coos and gurgles
✳ Moves eyes and head when the baby hears a sound
✳ Smiles and frowns

Six months

✳ Turns head when he/she hears a familiar voice
✳ Sings to themselves
✳ Laughs and chuckles

One year

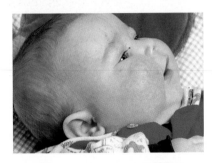

✳ Babbles e.g. da da
✳ Responds to own name
✳ Understands simple instructions

Eighteen months

✳ Can say about 6 words
✳ Understands more words than he/she can say
✳ Tries to sing
✳ Follows simple instructions
✳ Says and understands 'no'

2 years

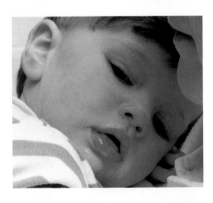

✳ Can say 50 or more words
✳ Begins to talk in simple sentences, e.g. Daddy up
✳ Likes to know names of objects
✳ Joins in with nursery rhymes

3 years

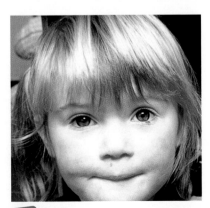

✳ Asks questions
✳ Listens to stories
✳ Can count to ten or more
✳ Has a good range of words
✳ Understands more
✳ Talks about things that have happened in the past

Childhood: 4–9 years

4 years

* Tells long stories
* Enjoys jokes
* Knows nursery rhymes and poems by heart
* Knows their own name and address
* Asks more questions
* Joins sentences with 'and' or 'but'

5 years

* Talks in the same way as an adult
* Loves to read and be told stories
* Asks the meaning of words
* Can predict results of actions
* Can carry on meaningful conversation with adult
* Talks about future events

7–9 years

* Is a fluent talker
* Vocabulary increases

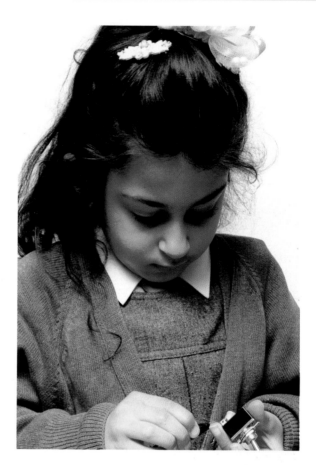

Adolescence, Adulthood and Later Life

* Vocabulary increases
* Understanding of new words increases
* Enjoys books, writing stories
* Talks to people of all ages

KEY TASKS

① What could you do to help a baby listen?

② How can you help an 18 month-old baby understand the meaning of new words?

③ How can you encourage a two year-old child to become interested in reading?

④ Describe an activity that you could do with a three year-old child which will help them to write.

⑤ Describe an activity, which will help a four year-old child listen more carefully.

⑥ How can you encourage a five year-old child to become better at talking?

⑦ How could you encourage an eight year-old child to write stories?

Memory Jogger

Look at the different stages of language development. Complete the table below.

1. Cries

2. Says short sentences e.g. daddy up

3. Frowns

4. Talks about future events

5. Babbling

6. Joins sentences with 'and' and 'but'

7. Smiles

8. Has approximately 50 words

9. Gurgles

10. Asks questions

11. Says 'no'

12. Talks in the same way as an adult

13. Uses complex sentences

14. Names objects

15. Listens to sounds

16. Tells short stories

17. Says 'don't', 'can't'

18. A few single words e.g. juice

19. Is able to follow instructions

20. Talks about things that have happened in the past

0 - 1 year	
1 - 3 years	
3 - 5 years	
5 - 8 years	

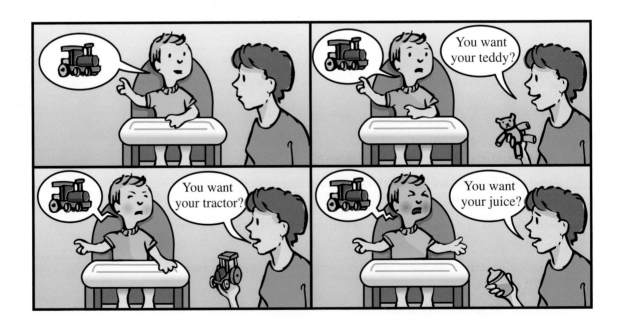

Why is language and communication important?

Language and communication are important because

✳ it lets us pass on information to other people
✳ we can talk about our feelings
✳ we can discuss problems.

Young children can become very frustrated because they want to tell you something but they cannot because they do not have the language needed.

We can communicate meaning in many different ways and not just through talking or writing.

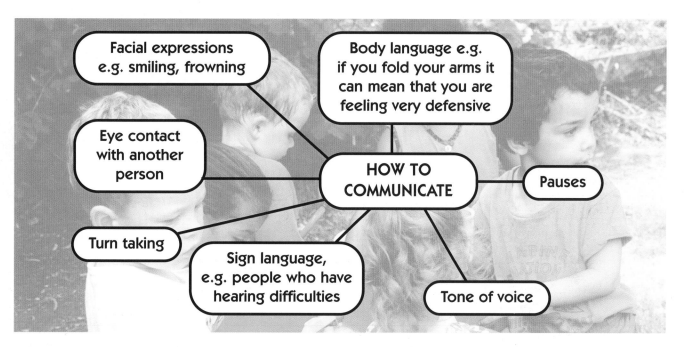

Young children learn to talk by:
✳ Listening to adults talking to them
✳ Listening to the sounds around them
✳ Practising new sounds
✳ Copying sounds made by others
✳ Learning what the sounds mean – young children understand more than they can say

SOCIAL DEVELOPMENT

Infancy: 0–3 years

Birth to three months

* Smile to adult
* Later on smiles to familiar adults and strangers
* Beginning to show temperament e.g. quiet baby, alert baby

Six months

* Uses fingers to feed themselves
* Gives toys to others
* Not so confident with strangers
* Upset with mother leaves room

One year

* Shy with strangers
* Like being with familiar people
* Enjoy mealtimes
* Help with daily routines, e.g. getting dressed

Eighteen months

* Happy to play on their own. This is known as solitary play.
* Want to be independent, e.g. feed themselves

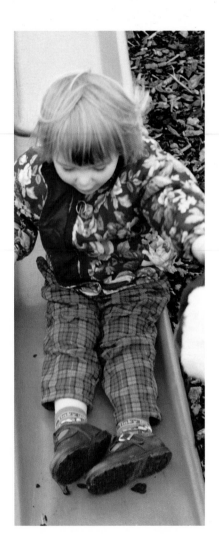

* May cling to familiar adult in strange surroundings
* Are developing a sense of identity

Two years

* Enjoy helping others
* Play alongside other children but not with them. This is known as parallel play.
* Not happy to share toys with other children
* Shows concern for other children who are crying or upset

Three years

* Happy to play with other children.
* Understands how to share
* Beginning to take turns
* Do not like to lose games
* Like to do things without help from others
* Beginning to understand the view point of other people
* Enjoy helping adults
* Becoming aware of being male or female

Childhood: 4–9 years

Four years

* Becoming more independent, e.g. able to wash themselves, dress and undress without help
* Show sensitivity towards others
* Can join in with games and then suddenly become aggressive
* Enjoys being with other children
* Enjoy planning play projects and playing with other children.

Five years

* Have definite likes and dislikes
* Are sympathetic when friends get hurt
* Choose their own friends

Six years

* Enjoy doing simple tasks around the house, e.g. tidying up bedroom
* Choose friends with similar interests and personalities
* Compare themselves to other people
* Enjoy playing games with other children

Seven–nine years

* Co-operates with friends
* Understands the need for rules
* Completely independent in dressing, washing, feeding skills
* Form important friendships
* Have a close friend usually their own sex
* Enjoys playing with other children who all have the same goal in mind. This is known as co-operative play.

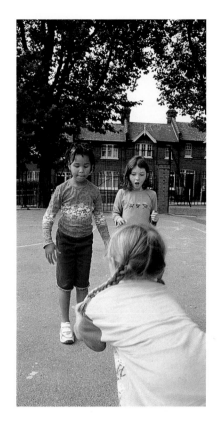

Between the age of 1 and 5 years children learn to play with other children. Most children go through the same stages of social play.

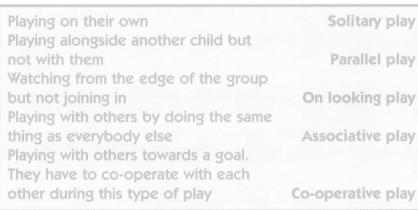

Playing on their own	Solitary play
Playing alongside another child but not with them	Parallel play
Watching from the edge of the group but not joining in	On looking play
Playing with others by doing the same thing as everybody else	Associative play
Playing with others towards a goal. They have to co-operate with each other during this type of play	Co-operative play

Adolescence: 10–18 years

* Need for individual identity
* Need to belong to a group
* Develop personal relationships with the opposite sex
* Begin to explore their sexuality

Adulthood: 19–65 years

✳ Similar to adolescence
✳ May experience marriage, divorce, parenthood
✳ Important to feel part of society

Later life: 65+

✳ Friendship groups may change
✳ Have different roles e.g. may become grandparents
✳ More leisure time to make new friends
✳ May be lonely and feel insecure

EMOTIONAL DEVELOPMENT

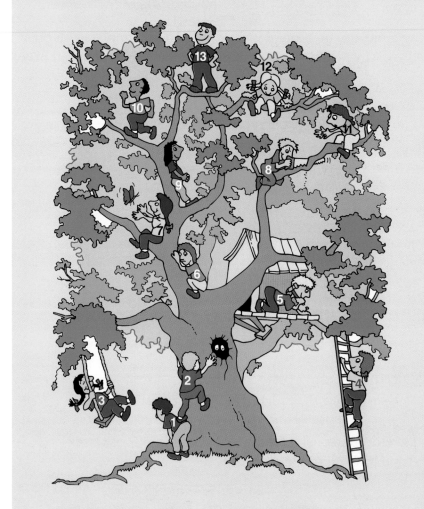

KEY TASKS

Look at the picture of the children in the tree. Describe how each child is feeling. Share your ideas in a small group.

As we get older we are able to control our emotions.

KEY TASKS

We all have positive emotions e.g. love, happy and negative emotions e.g. hate, frustration. Make a list of the positive and negative emotions that you feel.

Positive emotions	Negative emotions

Infancy: 0–3 Years

Birth to three months

* Is scared when not held firmly or hears sudden noises
* Cries if left on their own for too long
* Goes from being very happy to unhappy
* Wriggles body with pleasure

Six months

* Squeals with pleasure
* May be anxious towards strangers
* Usually friendly
* Is annoyed if a toy is taken away

One year

* Gets angry because they cannot do what they want to
* Is anxious if left on their own for some time
* No fear
* Very curious
* Friendly and confident

Two years

* May have tantrums
* Could have nightmares and irrational fears
* Loving and caring
* Tries to be independent

Three years

* Loving, friendly, co-operative
* Copies moods and attitudes of adults
* May have feelings of insecurity
* Becoming more self conscious and nervous

Childhood: 4–9 years

Four years

* Confident
* Some control over emotions
* Understands the standards of behaviour expected of them

Five years

* Self confident
* Boasts, shows off
* Wants to do well
* Some control over their emotions

Six years

* Swings from love to hate and back again
* Self centred, irritable and aggressive
* Can be loving, friendly and co-operative
* Find frustration and failure hard to cope with

Seven and eight years

* More stable than at six years
* Independent
* Enjoys being on their own
* Can be moody
* Can become over tired and irritable

Adolescence: 10–18 years

* Emotionally independent of adults
* Needs to be accepted by peer group
* Enjoys physical and intellectual tasks
* Good control of strong emotions

Adulthood: 19–65 years

* The menopause in women may cause changes in mood swings

Later Life: 65+

* May enjoy greater independence
* Enjoy retirement and opportunity to try new things
* May feel lonely and depressed
* May be unable to manage on their own and may lose some of their independence

Managing children's behaviour

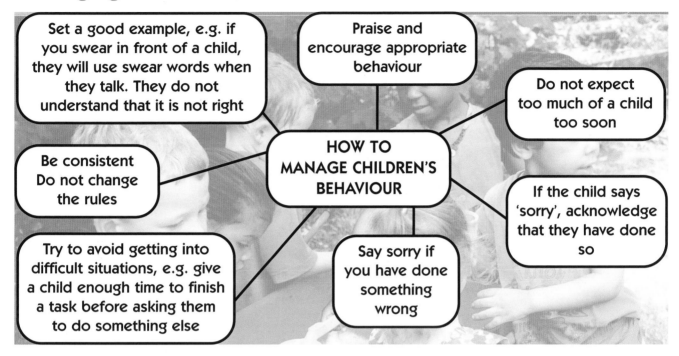

Set a good example, e.g. if you swear in front of a child, they will use swear words when they talk. They do not understand that it is not right

Praise and encourage appropriate behaviour

Do not expect too much of a child too soon

Be consistent Do not change the rules

HOW TO MANAGE CHILDREN'S BEHAVIOUR

If the child says 'sorry', acknowledge that they have done so

Try to avoid getting into difficult situations, e.g. give a child enough time to finish a task before asking them to do something else

Say sorry if you have done something wrong

Children are often difficult to manage when they are:

* Hungry
* Tired
* Lonely
* Worried
* Not well
* Bored
* Doing something that they know they cannot do

Adults find it difficult to manage children when they are:

* Not well
* Too busy
* Frustrated
* Feel they cannot cope, e.g. a crying baby
* Worried
* Tired
* Angry

2. WHAT AFFECTS THE GROWTH AND DEVELOPMENT OF A PERSON?

There are four main factors, which can affect growth and development:

1. Social and economic factors
2. Genetic factors
3. Health
4. Environment

1. Social and economic factors

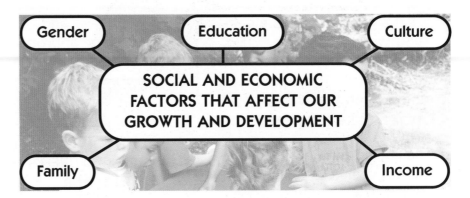

Gender

Although girls and boys should have the same opportunities, people still have different expectations of what girls and boys should do. There are very few men working in child care settings, for example.

Family

The family can teach children the skills, beliefs and values that will prepare them for later life. A parent may teach a child the difference between right and wrong.

Education

School and college can have a big impact on a person's development. Some children enjoy school but others hate it and do not feel that they have learned anything.

Culture

Our customs, religious beliefs and way of life can affect our development. Some religions forbid alcohol while some cultures arrange marriages for their daughters.

Income

The amount of money a family receives can affect their personal development. People who have a very low income and experience poverty are more likely to suffer from ill health. They are not so likely to get involved in leisure activities or attend college to improve their education.

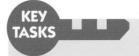

Choose **one** of the social factors above and think about the effect it has had on your development.

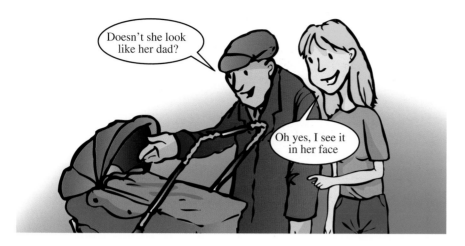

Genetic factors

All living things are able to pass on their own characteristic features from the parent to the child in the cells of the body, e.g. colour of eyes or hair. We get our characteristics from our parents. Our parents get their characteristics from their parents.

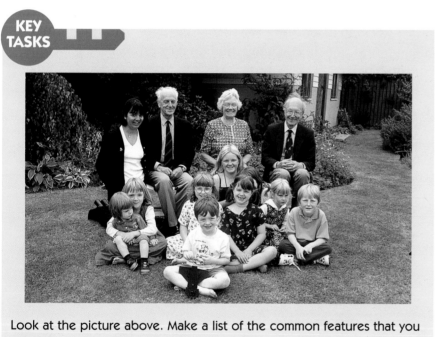

Look at the picture above. Make a list of the common features that you can see.

The characteristics that we inherit are carried in our genes. You may have included colour of hair and eyes, height, shape of different parts of the body in your answer.

Illnesses can also be passed on from one generation to another through genes, e.g. cystic fibrosis.

Health

A healthy and balanced diet ensures that we grow and develop in an appropriate way. Too much or too little food can affect our health.

Physical exercise is also important for our growth and development. Adults should be involved in energetic activity at least three times a week.

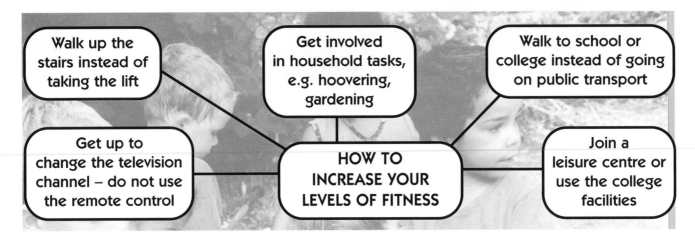

Walk up the stairs instead of taking the lift

Get up to change the television channel – do not use the remote control

Get involved in household tasks, e.g. hoovering, gardening

HOW TO INCREASE YOUR LEVELS OF FITNESS

Walk to school or college instead of going on public transport

Join a leisure centre or use the college facilities

Stress can also affect our growth and development. It can cause unhappiness, loneliness, abuse and dietary problems e.g. people eat too much or eat very little.

Environment

The environment that we grow up in can have a big impact on our growth and development.

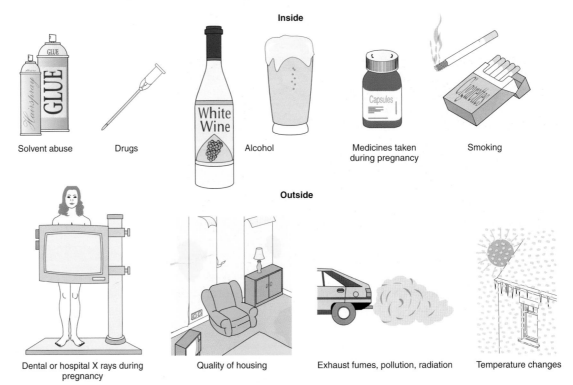

Inside

Solvent abuse   Drugs   Alcohol   Medicines taken during pregnancy   Smoking

Outside

Dental or hospital X rays during pregnancy   Quality of housing   Exhaust fumes, pollution, radiation   Temperature changes

What can affect the development of the body?

Drugs

Any drugs may affect the growth and development of the baby including street or illegal drugs. When we talk about 'drugs' it usually refers to a habit-forming substance e.g. ecstasy, heroin, cannabis or solvents.

The baby suffers withdrawal symptoms if the mother takes drugs

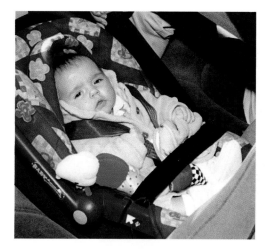

The baby may be born with a physical or learning disability if the mother takes drugs

Cocaine, crack, heroin, amphetamines and cannabis are known to affect the baby.

Alcohol

Alcohol is a type of drug. When a pregnant mother has a drink the baby takes in alcohol as well. Regular drinking by the mother can affect the growth and development of the baby or may cause a miscarriage. Light, occasional drinking i.e. one or two units once or twice a week, is not likely to do the baby any harm.

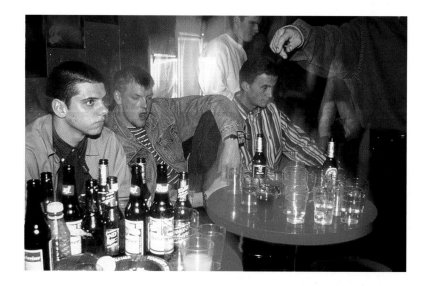

Excessive drinking can also affect the development of teenagers and adults. The short-term effects of drinking too much alcohol are headaches, sleeping problems and poor concentration.

Smoking

Smoking can seriously damage your health and your baby's.

Chemicals pass from the mother's lungs into the blood stream and then into the uterus The chemicals enter the baby's blood stream when they pass over the placenta

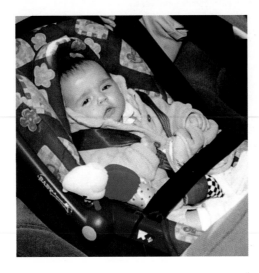

Nicotine will make the baby's heart beat faster

Cot death (Sudden Infant Death Syndrome) is more likely in babies who have been exposed to tobacco smoke

Heavy smokers are more likely to have a miscarriage

Carbon monoxide will affect the oxygen levels in the baby

KEY TASKS

Collect leaflets and booklets that give information to parents about the effects of drugs, alcohol and smoking on pregnant women. Use the information to make a poster explaining the effects on the growth and development of the baby.

Solvent abuse

'Using ordinary household products like cigarette lighter refills, aerosols, glue, petrol and other products to get 'high' is known as solvent or volatile substance abuse (VSA). In an average home there are over 30 abusable products.'
Source: Resolv 1998

Source: Unknown

TEST YOURSELF

① List the **five** main life stages.

② John is 83 years old. What life stage is this?

③ Shakila is 10 years old. What life stage is this?

④ Give **two** other names for 'adolescence'.

⑤ Match the statement about child development to the appropriate age.

AGE OF CHILD	STATEMENT ABOUT CHILD DEVELOPMENT	
Newborn	c	f
Infant	i	b
2 year old	j	d
5 year old	a	e
8 year old	g	h
12 year old	k	l

a) Can skip with a rope and ride a two-wheel bicycle

b) Shy with strangers

c) Can identify the smell of the mother's milk

d) Finds it difficult to share toys

e) Can dress without help from an adult. May still need help to tie shoelaces.

f) Has several reflexes, including the grasp and sucking reflex

g) Prefers the company of his/her own sex.

h) Like being in groups of children of their own age.

i) Uses senses to learn about their world

j) Has tantrums if frustrated

k) Is very fashion conscious

⑥ What can affect the growth and development of a child? Give **three** examples.

⑦ How can smoking affect the growth and development of a baby? Give **two** examples?

⑧ List **three** social and economic factors that may affect the development of a person.

⑨ What are the physical differences between an adolescent boy and adolescent girl? Give **three** different examples.

⑩ What physical changes happen to a person in old age? Give **four** examples.

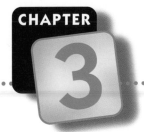

Food and Nutrition

* Healthy eating
* Preparing and presenting food for children
* Feeding babies
* The influence of different religions and cultures on diet

1. HEALTHY EATING

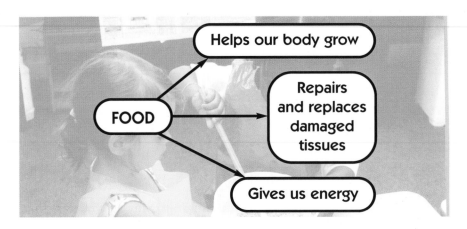

What is meant by a 'healthy balanced diet'?

There are no 'healthy' or 'unhealthy' foods. There are 'healthy' and 'unhealthy' diets. Healthy eating is achieved when we have a balanced and varied healthy diet.

A healthy balanced diet should have:

* fruit and vegetables
* bread, other cereals and potatoes
* milk and other dairy products
* fatty and sugary foods
* meat, fish and alternatives.

Most adults should eat foods which contain less fat and less sugar. No matter what you do, you still need to have the right

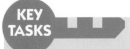

KEY TASKS

Make a list of the food you ate yesterday. Do you think you had a healthy balanced diet that day? What could you have eaten that would have made it better?

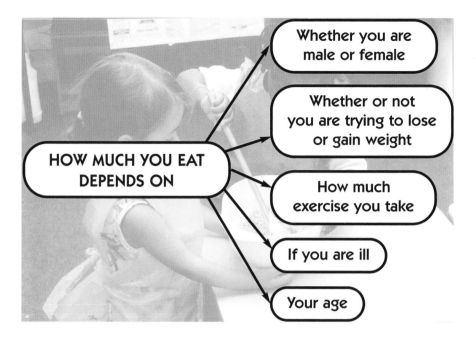

Whether you are
male or female

Whether or not
you are trying to lose
or gain weight

**HOW MUCH YOU EAT
DEPENDS ON**

How much
exercise you take

If you are ill

Your age

proportions of each different type of food to be healthy.

A balanced diet

Healthy eating is important for everyone. A healthy balanced diet
is good for you because it:

* gives your body all the nutrients it needs to grow and
  develop properly
* gives your body the energy to live life to the full
* can improve your concentration
* helps you to fight infection and keeps you well
* helps to protect you against long-term illness, e.g. heart
  disease, strokes and cancer.

A poor diet can result in:

* obesity or anorexia
* heart disease in later life
* anaemia resulting from insufficient iron intake
* dental decay from eating too much sugar
* poor resistance to infection resulting from lack of vitamins

Memory Jogger

① What does food do for us? Give three
  examples.
② Name the five types of food that give us a
  balanced diet.
③ What happens if you do not eat a balanced diet? Give
  three examples.

and minerals

✳ inadequate build up of bone density resulting from insufficient calcium intakes, along with too little physical activity, which can lead to the risk of osteoporosis (brittle bones) in later life.

The main nutrients and where they are found

What is a nutrient?

Each piece of food that we eat is made up of different nutrients, i.e. chemicals. After we have eaten a piece of food the nutrients are absorbed.

The body uses nutrients to

✳ help it to grow,
✳ be repaired and
✳ keep our body tissue healthy.

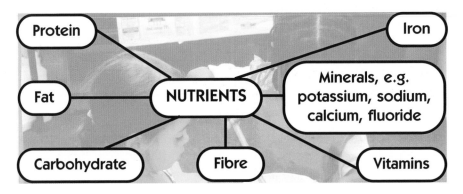

Protein • Iron • Fat • NUTRIENTS • Minerals, e.g. potassium, sodium, calcium, fluoride • Carbohydrate • Fibre • Vitamins

Memory Jogger

Make up a sentence to help you to remember the names of the different nutrients using the first letter of each word to help you. For example:

P	(protein)	people
I	(iron)	in
C	(carbohydrate)	caravans
M	(minerals)	might
F	(fibre)	feel
V	(vitamin)	very
F	(fat)	fat

You can use the letters in any order you like and you can make the sentence as silly as you like – as long as it helps you to remember the main nutrients that are present in food.

What do nutrients do?

Protein is needed for the growth and repair of our body cells	Iron helps to produce haemoglobin which takes oxygen around in the blood	Carbohydrate gives us energy and helps us to digest our food. 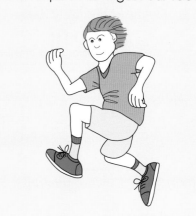
Different minerals do different things e.g. Calcium helps to form strong bones and teeth Fluoride helps strengthen the enamel on our teeth Phosphorous works with calcium to build strong bones and teeth Fat gives us energy. It protects our vital organs e.g. heart and helps to absorb vitamins A, D, E and K. It also gives us warmth.	Fibre adds bulk to food and helps to prevent constipation 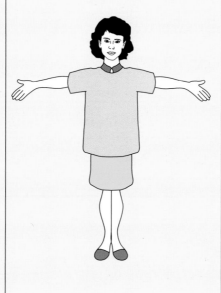	Different vitamins have different functions e.g. Vitamin A is important for good eye sight Vitamin B1 keeps our nervous system healthy Vitamin B2 is important for healthy skin Vitamin C is essential for our body tissue Vitamin D works with calcium and phosphorous to give us strong bones and teeth

WHAT ARE THE BEST SOURCES OF MINERALS AND VITAMINS?

VITAMIN A	Liver Carrots Spinach Watercress Red peppers Mango Dried apricots	ZINC	Liver Kidney Lean meat Corned beef Nuts
VITAMIN B	Liver Pork, ham, bacon Breakfast cereals Chicken	IRON	Breakfast cereals Liver Dried fruit, e.g. apricots, prunes, raisins
VITAMIN C	Blackcurrants Oranges and orange juice Strawberries Green and red peppers	CALCIUM	Spinach Sardines Cheese Tofu
VITAMIN D	Breakfast cereals Pilchards Herring Sardines Tuna Canned salmon Egg	FIBRE	Whole grain Whole wheat Branflakes Wholemeal bread Chick peas Baked beans Lentils Dried prunes
SODIUM CHLORIDE	Salt Fish Meat Processed foods		

KEY TASKS

Design a poster, which shows the main nutrients and where they are found.

Memory Jogger

① How many main nutrients are there?
② List the main nutrients. (If you made up a rhyme, you should be able to do it from memory.)
③ Which nutrients help to make our teeth and bones strong?
④ What does fat do?
⑤ Which nutrient is needed for the growth and repair of our body cells?
⑥ Which nutrients give us energy?

EIGHT STEPS TO A HEALTHY DIET

✳ Enjoy your food.
✳ Eat a variety of different foods.
✳ Eat the right amount to be a healthy weight.
✳ Eat plenty of foods rich in starch and fibre.
✳ Do not eat too much fat.
✳ Do not eat sugary foods too often.
✳ Look after the vitamins and minerals in your food.
✳ If you drink alcohol, keep within sensible limits.

Ministry of Agriculture, Fisheries and Food 1990

WHAT SHOULD CHILDREN EAT EACH DAY?

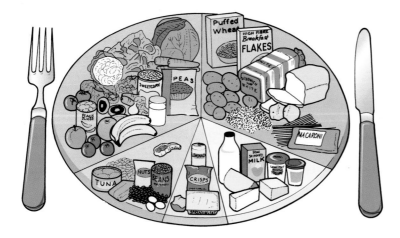

We gain energy from the food we eat. Children need different amounts of energy depending on how old they are. Energy in food is measured in Kcal (kilocalories).

The table below shows the average energy requirements in kilocalories (Kcals) that a child needs each day.

AGE	BOYS	GIRLS
	Kcals	Kcals
1–3 years	1230	1165
4–6 years	1715	1545
7–10 years	1970	1740
11–14 years	2220	1845
15–18 years	2755	2100

Children and adults will gain weight if they eat more calories than their body needs each day.

Children should be encouraged to eat five child-sized portions of fruit and vegetables each day

Children should have a diet rich in iron, e.g. meat, fish and poultry. Children who do not eat meat should have cereals, pulses, fruit and vegetables

Their diet should have enough energy (calories) to ensure healthy grow and development

Children should drink water if they are thirsty

WHAT SHOULD CHILDREN AGED BETWEEN 1 AND 5 YEARS OF AGE EAT AND DRINK?

Starchy foods, e.g. potatoes, pasta, bread and rice are better sources of energy than sugary foods

Diluted fruit juice is a good source of Vitamin C

Whole cow milk is a good drink for children from 12 months of age

Planning a healthy diet for young children
Memory Jogger

① How many portions of fruit and vegetables should a child eat each day?
② What can a child eat if they do not eat meat?
③ What starch food can a child eat?
④ What can if child drink if they are thirsty? Give three examples.
⑤ What do calories give?

Breakfast

TYPE OF FOOD	NUTRIENTS	HOW MUCH PER DAY
FRUIT AND VEGETABLES	Vitamin C Iron Calcium Fibre Some carbohydrate	4 or 5 portions each day
BREAD, OTHER CEREALS AND POTATOES	Carbohydrate Fibre Some calcium and iron Vitamin B	All meals should include bread, cereal or potato
MILK AND OTHER DAIRY PRODUCTS	Calcium Protein Vitamin A, B and D	Children need up to one pint of milk each day
FATTY AND OTHER SUGARY FOODS	Vitamins A lot of fat, sugar and salt	Eat as little as possible
MEAT, FISH AND OTHER ALTERNATIVES	Iron Protein Vitamins Zinc and magnesium	Two portions should be eaten each day. Vegetarians can eat grains, pulses and seeds.

Breakfast is considered to be the most important meal of the day. If children and adults do not have anything for breakfast they often are tempted to snack on foods that are high in fat or sugar during the day. Breakfast foods are a good source of fibre, minerals and vitamins.

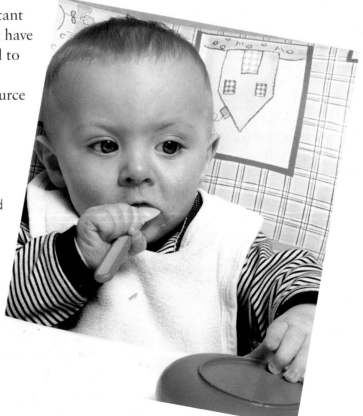

Adults working with children should:
* Encourage the child to get up early enough to have time for breakfast.
* Eat breakfast with the child to set a good example.
* Provide bread, cereals or fruit and avoid sugary foods or drinks.
* Provide a healthy snack for the child to eat during the day.

Mid-morning or mid-afternoon snack (if required)

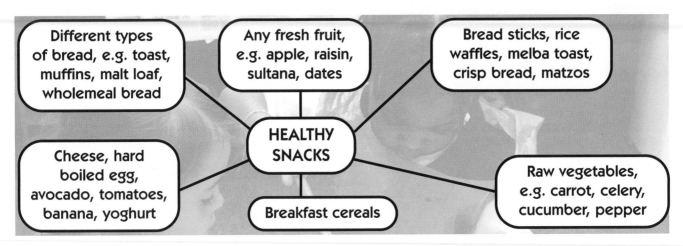

Different types of bread, e.g. toast, muffins, malt loaf, wholemeal bread

Any fresh fruit, e.g. apple, raisin, sultana, dates

Bread sticks, rice waffles, melba toast, crisp bread, matzos

HEALTHY SNACKS

Cheese, hard boiled egg, avocado, tomatoes, banana, yoghurt

Breakfast cereals

Raw vegetables, e.g. carrot, celery, cucumber, pepper

Packed lunches

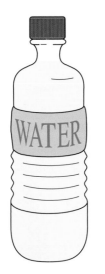

Children often have a packed lunch rather than a nursery or school lunch. Packed lunches should be varied and healthy.

A healthy packed lunch could have:

* bread, pitta bread, chapatti or rice cakes
* fish, meat or an alternative, e.g. cheese, egg, peanut butter, houmous
* two portions of fruit and/or vegetables, e.g carrot sticks, celery, dried fruit.

Other foods could include yoghurt, breadsticks, sunflower seeds etc. Crisps are very high in fat and salt so should not be put in the lunch box.

Drinks

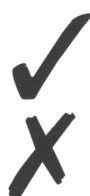

* Water
* Milk
* Milkshakes
* Smoothies (liquid yoghurt)

* Fizzy drinks
* Squash
* Fruit drinks
* Sports drinks

Evening meal

The evening meal should not be eaten too late in the day, as it does not give the body time to digest properly.

KEY TASKS

Pasta, sweet corn and sausage salad

Wholemeal muffin

Kiwi fruit

Fruit juice or sugar-free drink

Is this a healthy lunch for a six year-old child? Give reasons for your answer.

KEY TASKS

Plan a midday meal for a three year–old child. List the nutrients for each food that you use.

2. PREPARING AND PRESENTING FOOD FOR CHLDREN

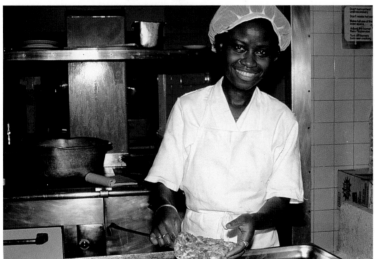

Preparing food in a safe and hygienic way

✳ Always wash your hands really well before you touch food.
✳ Put a blue waterproof dressing on cuts.
✳ Tie hair back out of the way.
✳ Clean all surfaces with disinfectant.
✳ Have different colours of chopping boards.
✳ Use different boards for meat and vegetables.
✳ All cutlery, crockery and cooking utensils should be washed after use in hot soapy water, rinsed and dried thoroughly before storing.
✳ Rubbish bins should be emptied and cleaned regularly.
✳ The kitchen should be free from flies.

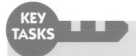

KEY TASKS

Design a poster, which explains how to handle food in a safe and hygienic way.

KEY TASKS

This adult is not preparing food in a safe way. Find five errors and describe what she should be doing.

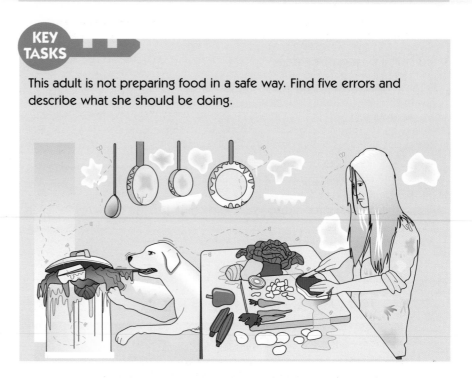

Presenting food to young children

Meal times are an important part of the child's day. The food should be presented in an attractive way, which will encourage the child to eat.

① Know what the child likes and does not like.

② Ask the child what they would like for the meal.

③ Plan the meal so that the child has something from each of the five food groups.

④ Make sure that the food is easy to eat, e.g. not too difficult to chew.

⑤ Encourage the child's independence by giving them food that they can eat themselves, e.g. small pieces.

⑥ Give suitable cutlery, e.g. a young child may need to use a spoon instead of a fork, some children will use chopsticks.

⑦ Present the food in an interesting way, e.g. different shapes of pasta.

⑧ Do not make the portions too big. An older child may be allowed to choose how much they want to eat.

⑨ Praise the child through the meal.

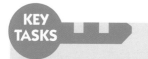
KEY TASKS

Peter is three years old. He does not enjoy mealtimes and will only eat chips. What could you do to make mealtimes more enjoyable?

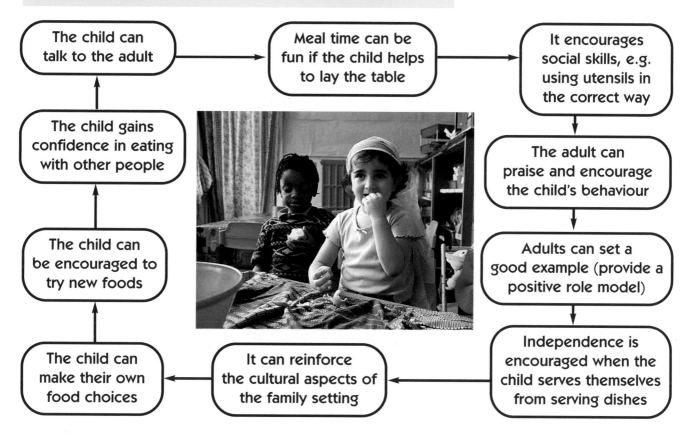

The child can talk to the adult → Meal time can be fun if the child helps to lay the table → It encourages social skills, e.g. using utensils in the correct way

The child gains confidence in eating with other people

The adult can praise and encourage the child's behaviour

The child can be encouraged to try new foods

Adults can set a good example (provide a positive role model)

The child can make their own food choices ← It can reinforce the cultural aspects of the family setting ← Independence is encouraged when the child serves themselves from serving dishes

3. FEEDING BABIES

Young babies can either be:

* breast-fed or
* bottle-fed using formulas based on cow's milk.

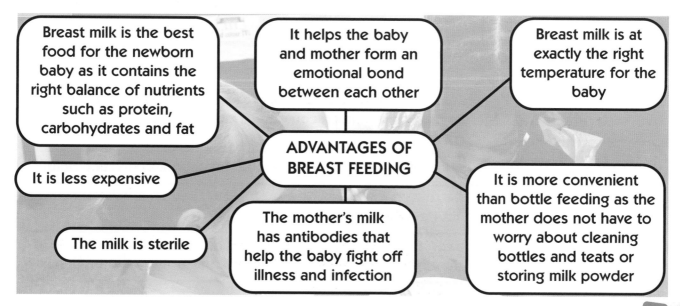

Breast milk is the best food for the newborn baby as it contains the right balance of nutrients such as protein, carbohydrates and fat

It helps the baby and mother form an emotional bond between each other

Breast milk is at exactly the right temperature for the baby

ADVANTAGES OF BREAST FEEDING

It is less expensive

The milk is sterile

The mother's milk has antibodies that help the baby fight off illness and infection

It is more convenient than bottle feeding as the mother does not have to worry about cleaning bottles and teats or storing milk powder

Both methods of feeding have advantages and disadvantages.

In the first few days of the baby's life, they will be fed regularly. They do not need a lot of food but they enjoy sucking and being close to the mother.

However, babies get hungry very quickly. Over 24 hours, they will want to be fed between ten and twelve times. The more the baby sucks, the more milk the mother is able to produce.

After a few weeks the baby begins to get into a feeding routine. Most babies will want to be fed about six times over 24 hours.

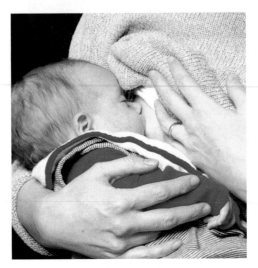 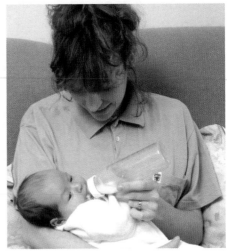

When the baby is about three months old, the night-time feed is no longer required. However this does vary from one baby to another.

Most mothers will breast-feed until the baby is between four to six months. Some mothers stop earlier if they want to return to work, while others breast-feed for longer.

Some mothers do not breast-feed their babies for a variety of different reasons.

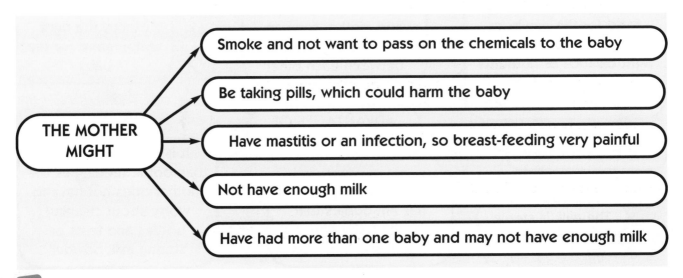

THE MOTHER MIGHT

Smoke and not want to pass on the chemicals to the baby

Be taking pills, which could harm the baby

Have mastitis or an infection, so breast-feeding very painful

Not have enough milk

Have had more than one baby and may not have enough milk

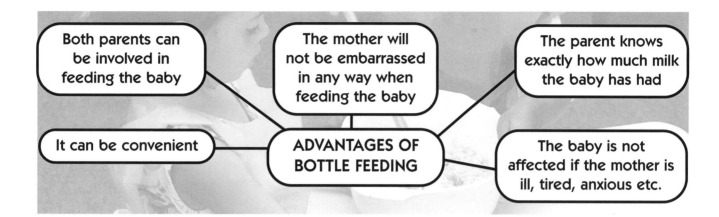

Both parents can be involved in feeding the baby

It can be convenient

The mother will not be embarrassed in any way when feeding the baby

ADVANTAGES OF BOTTLE FEEDING

The parent knows exactly how much milk the baby has had

The baby is not affected if the mother is ill, tired, anxious etc.

Preparing feeds

Ordinary cow's milk should not be given to babies under the age of six months and preferably not under the age of nine months.

It is very important that the bottle and any other equipment you use has been sterilised.

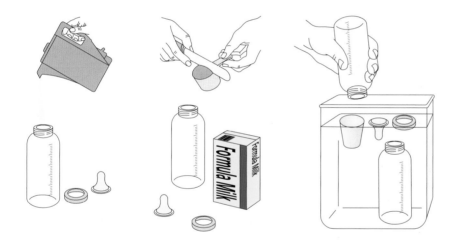

Before you start, you will need:

* a container for sterilising the bottle in
* bottle
* a teat with the right size of hole for the baby (if the hole is too big the baby could choke – if the hole is too small the baby will swallow a lot of air and have trouble with wind)
* large plastic jug and a plastic stirrer
* sterilising tablets or liquid.

Preparing the bottle

Before you start you will need:

* milk formula
* boiled water
* a plastic straight edged knife
* glass jug
* feeding bottle and teat.

Then you should:

① Wash your hands before you begin.

② Make sure that all the equipment has been sterilised.

③ Follow the instructions on the milk formula packet.

④ Fill the jug with the right amount of hot water.

⑤ Add the correct amount of powder. You could make the baby ill if you do not use the correct amount.

⑥ **Never add salt or sugar.**

⑦ Stir the liquid to make sure there are no lumps.

⑧ Fill the feeding bottle.

⑨ Put the teat and the teat protector on to the bottle.

Sometimes you can make the milk formula in the feeding bottle.

① Store the bottle in the refrigerator until you are ready to use it.

② Warm the bottle in a jug of hot water or a baby warmer. Do not use a microwave because some of the milk may be too hot.

③ Check the temperature of the milk before you give it to the baby. Drip a little of the milk onto the inside of your wrist to find out if it is too hot or too cold.

④ Wash your hands again before you start to feed the baby.

When you feed the baby:

① Hold the baby in the same way as you would hold a baby who was being breast-fed.

② Make sure that the hole in the teat is not blocked.

③ Tilt the bottle to make sure that there is no gap between the teat and the liquid.

④ Keep the teat full of milk.

⑤ Talk to the baby and keep eye contact as you are feeding it.

⑥ Stop feeding the baby every so often and 'wind' the baby. Air can get trapped in the baby's stomach and it can be sore.

⑦ Never leave the baby on their own with the bottle in their mouth. The baby could choke. The baby could also be swallowing too much air.

⑧ Do not rush the baby. It will take time.

When you have fed the baby you should:

✳ change the baby
✳ make sure the baby is safe and happy
✳ Clear away and sterilise the equipment

Weaning

Weaning is when the baby starts to eat solid food.

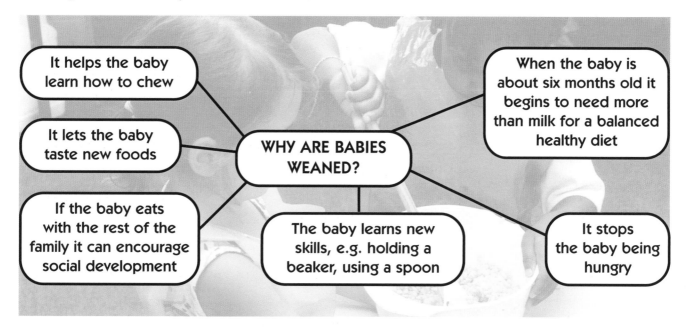

It helps the baby learn how to chew

It lets the baby taste new foods

If the baby eats with the rest of the family it can encourage social development

WHY ARE BABIES WEANED?

When the baby is about six months old it begins to need more than milk for a balanced healthy diet

The baby learns new skills, e.g. holding a beaker, using a spoon

It stops the baby being hungry

What should a child aged 4–12 months eat?

4–6 MONTHS	6–8 MONTHS	9–12 MONTHS
You can give: Puréed fruit and vegetables Thin porridge made from oats or rice meal Finely puréed dhal or lentils	**You can add:** A wider range of puréed fruits and vegetables Wheat based foods, e.g. mashed Weetabix Egg yolk, well cooked Small sized beans such as aduki beans, cooked soft Pieces of ripe banana Cooked rice Citrus fruits Soft summer fruits Pieces of bread	**You can add:** An increasingly wide range of foods with a variety of textures and flavours Cow's milk Fromage frais Yoghurt Pieces of fish Soft cooked beans Pasta A variety of breads Pieces of meat from a casserole
How: Offer the food on the tip of a clean finger or on the tip of a plastic teaspoon	**How:** On a teaspoon	**How:** On a spoon or as finger food
Why: The start of moving from milk to solids	**Why:** At the end of the milk feed	**Why:** To encourage independence
Not yet: Cow's milk Citrus fruit Soft summer fruits Eggs, nuts, salt, sugar, fatty food Spinach Wheat Spices	**Not yet:** Cow's milk Chilli or chilli powder Egg whites Nuts, salt, sugar, fatty food	**Not yet:** Whole nuts Salt, sugar, fatty foods

Source: The Nursery Food Book. Mary Whiting and Tim Lobstein (1992)

KEY TASKS

Working in small groups, find out what processed baby food tastes like. You could use the chart on page 103 to help you.

MAKE AND FLAVOUR OF BABY FOOD	DESCRIBE WHAT IT LOOKS LIKE	DESCRIBE WHAT IT SMELLS LIKE	COMMENT ON THE FLAVOUR. DOES IT TASTE LIKE THE REAL THING?	MARKS OUT OF 10
e.g. Boots Carrot and potato				

4. THE INFLUENCE OF DIFFERENT RELIGIONS AND CULTURES ON DIET

When preparing food for young children it is essential to take account of their religious and cultural needs.

	JEWISH	HINDI	SIKH	MUSLIM	BUDDHIST	RASTAFARIAN
EGGS	No blood spots	Some	Yes	Yes	Some	Some
MILK/YOGHURT	Not with meat	Yes	Yes	Yes	Yes	Some
CHEESE	Not with meat	Some	Some	Possibly	Yes	Some
CHICKEN	Kosher	Some	Some	Halal	No	Some
MUTTON/LAMB	Kosher	Some	Yes	Halal	No	Some
BEEF AND BEEF PRODUCTS	Kosher	No	No	Halal	No	Some
PORK AND PORK PRODUCTS	No	No	Rarely	No	No	No
FISH	With fins, backbones and scales	With fins, backbones and scales	Some	Some	Some	Yes
SHELLFISH	No	Some	Some	Some	No	No
BUTTER/GHEE	Kosher	Some	Some	Some	No	Some
LARD	No	No	No	No	No	No
CEREAL FOODS	Yes	Yes	Yes	Yes	Yes	Yes
NUTS/PULSES	Yes	Yes	Yes	Yes	Yes	Yes
FRUITS/VEGETABLES	Yes	Yes	Yes	Yes	Yes	Yes
FASTING	Yes	Yes	Yes	Yes	Yes	Yes

Source: Eating well for looked after children and young people 2001

There are a wide variety of different cultures represented in child care settings and it is important to learn about each one.

Some religions do not allow their followers to eat certain foods.

Strict Hindus and Sikhs will not eat eggs, meat, fish and some fats.

Some Rastafarians are vegan i.e they do not eat animal products.

Fasting is unlikely to apply to young children.

Memory Jogger

True or false

Use the table on page 103 to help you to answer the questions.

1. Hindus eat no meat and drink no alcohol. Many devout Hindus are vegetarian.
2. Muslims do not eat pork or pork products. They do not drink alcohol.
3. Jewish people do not eat pork or shellfish. All other meat must be kosher. Milk and meat are not used together in cooking.
4. Rastafarians are usually vegetarian. They do not eat pork.
5. Vegetarians do not eat meat and may not eat other animal products.
6. Vegans do not eat any animal products.

Food allergies

Some people react in different ways to different foods for a number of different reasons.

Foods which can cause allergies

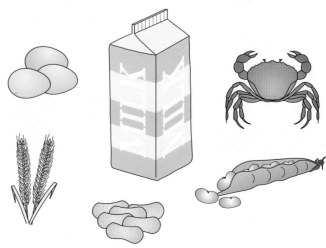

A bad reaction to food can cause headaches, indigestion, diarrhoea, aches and pains, vomiting, itchy rashes and wheezing.

Allergic reactions to food

Severe reactions to some foods can be life-threatening, e.g. peanuts. To help prevent peanut allergy, pregnant and breast feeding women who have allergies (e.g. asthma, eczema or hay fever) in their family are advised to avoid peanuts and peanut products to reduce the risk of their children developing a peanut allergy later in life.

Food colourings such as tartrazine (E102) can cause problems for children. They can become hyperactive or have an asthma attack.

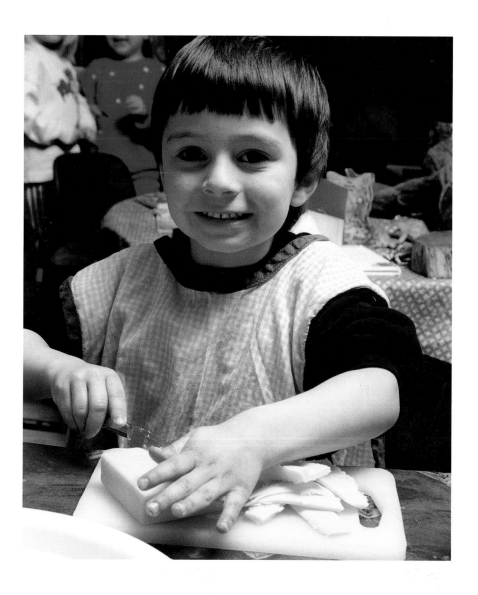

TEST YOURSELF

1. What should a healthy balanced diet have in it?

2. Why is it important to have a balanced diet?

3. What is a nutrient?

4. What do nutrients do for our bodies? Draw a line from the nutrient to the best answer.

Nutrient	What it does for our body
Protein	Gives us warmth
Iron	Strong bones and teeth
Carbohydrate	Repairs body cells
Fibre	Good eye sight
Vitamin	Takes oxygen round the blood
Fat	Gives bulk to our food
Minerals	Gives us energy

5. What should children aged between one and five years eat and drink? Give **three** examples.

6. Why is breakfast an important meal? Give **three** reasons.

7. Why are meal times important? Give **three** reasons.

8. Name two ways to feed a baby. Give **two** advantages for each method.

9. What does 'weaning' mean? When should it start?

10. What food could a child be allergic to? Give **three** examples.

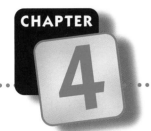

CHAPTER 4

Health and Safety

✳ Personal hygiene
✳ How to stop infection spreading
✳ Storing and handling foods safely
✳ A safe environment
✳ First aid

1. PERSONAL HYGIENE

People who are good to work with …

Wash regularly
Have a shower or bath every day, if possible. To look and feel good you should wash regularly and eat a healthy diet.

Use deodorants
Use light scented or non-perfumed anti-perspirants to reduce perspiration. Avoid highly scented deodorants, which hide body odours.

Care for their teeth
Brush your teeth regularly to avoid bad breath and poor teeth. Use floss and visit your dentist regularly. When working, avoid eating foods that are likely to leave you with an unpleasant breath, e.g. garlic or onions.

Wear clean clothes
Change your underwear every day.
Make sure your clothes are washed well.

Care for their hair
Your hair should be clean and neat when you are working. Long hair should be tied back, particularly if you are working with young children who are prone to lice and nits. Wash your hair frequently. Do not comb or brush your hair in the kitchen or around other people.

Care for their feet
Wash your feet well and make sure you dry them well. Use foot powders if necessary. Wear comfortable shoes. Make sure your tights or socks are clean.

Have clean hands
Wash your hands well after going to the toilet to avoid infection. Keep your nails short and clean. If you use nail varnish, make sure it is in good condition and not flaking off. Avoid too much jewellery.

A friend in your group has not washed for a week. Their hair is greasy, their nails are dirty and their clothes have obviously not been washed for a long time. Others in the group are either avoiding the person or they are giggling behind their back.

① As a friend, how do you feel about the situation?

② How would you tell your friend that they have a problem without upsetting them?

③ How do you think your friend will feel when you talk to them about the problem?

Working in small groups, role-play the situation. One person should take on the role of the friend who has the personal hygiene problem. One or two people could take on the role of the friends trying to help. One person should watch what happens and take notes during the role-play. They should be prepared to talk about what they have seen during the role-play.

What is infection?

✳ Germs go into the body through our mouth, nose, eyes, ears and cuts. They begin to increase in number.

✳ Our body reacts to the germs and uses different ways to destroy them.

✳ We become ill. The germs react to our body and our body reacts to the germs.

Not all germs cause illness in humans.

Why do you think children are more prone to infection than adults? What other age groups are more vulnerable?

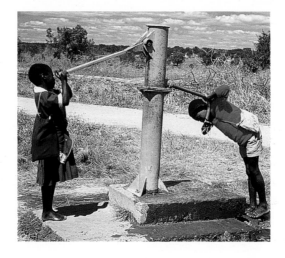

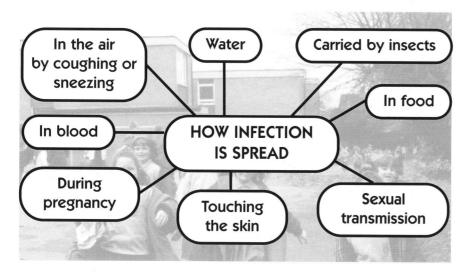

In the air by coughing or sneezing

Water

Carried by insects

In food

In blood

HOW INFECTION IS SPREAD

During pregnancy

Touching the skin

Sexual transmission

2. PREVENTING THE SPREAD OF INFECTION

ALWAYS WASH YOUR HANDS

✳ After you have used the toilet.
✳ Before you handle food.
✳ After blowing your nose or sneezing.
✳ After you have handled animals.
✳ After you have handled waste products of any kind, e.g. changing young children's nappies.
✳ Before you carry out first aid, if possible and after you have helped the child.

PERSONAL HYGIENE

✳ Never use other people's towels, hair brushes or toothbrushes.
✳ Children's personal items should be named when they are at playgroup or in the nursery, e.g. toothbrush, towel, flannel.

IMMUNISATION

✳ Children can be immunised against infectious diseases using a vaccine, e.g. MMR – one injection is given to help prevent measles, mumps and rubella.

DISPOSING OF WASTE PRODUCTS

✳ Always wear disposable gloves if handling waste products or carrying out hygiene routines, e.g. changing nappies.
✳ Nappies should be wrapped in special sealed bags.
✳ A separate bucket should be used for disposing of nappies, cotton wool, tissues etc.

ISOLATION

✳ If someone is suffering from an infectious illness they will be put into a room on their own to prevent the illness spreading to other people.

DISINFECTION

✳ Toys and play equipment can be disinfected to prevent infection spreading.

Did you know?

Our body has a natural ability to resist infection.

When we 'catch' an infectious disease, our body produces antibodies, which will help to destroy the germs. They also help to prevent you catching that illness again.

Memory Jogger

Can you spell all the words that you have found in the wordsearch?

Infection	Insects	Sex	Sneezing	Coughing
Pregnancy	Food	Skin	Water	Immunisation
Blood	Vaccine	Isolation		

I	M	M	U	N	I	S	A	T	I	O	N
N	L	Z	B	F	T	B	B	A	B	P	E
F	T	P	I	S	O	L	A	T	I	O	N
E	O	A	D	L	O	T	F	Y	J	F	I
C	G	O	H	O	Z	W	C	M	N	W	G
T	F	S	D	H	L	N	B	Q	I	L	N
I	W	W	Q	I	A	V	E	I	K	B	I
O	A	T	I	N	S	E	C	T	S	G	Z
N	T	B	G	M	R	A	J	W	P	R	E
L	E	E	L	Q	I	G	K	R	X	N	E
E	R	V	A	C	C	I	N	E	R	E	N
P	C	O	U	G	H	I	N	G	A	T	S

3. STORING AND HANDLING FOODS SAFELY

Food needs to be carefully looked after to avoid food poisoning. You can help to prevent food poisoning by:

✷ Choosing suitable foods in the shops
✷ Storing it carefully
✷ Cooking it appropriately

'Use by' dates

It is illegal for shops to sell food that has passed its 'use by' date.

'Use by' dates are put on perishable foods to give a definite date to use the food by. The food may look and smell fresh but there is no guarantee that it is. If the 'use by' date has passed the food should be thrown away.

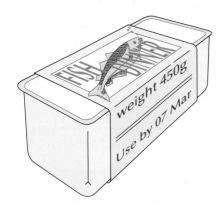

FISH DINNER
weight 450g
Use by 07 Mar

Storage instructions will also appear on foods. If you do not follow these instructions, the food may not last as long as the 'use by' date.

'Best before' dates

If food can be kept safely for a longer period of time, it will have a 'best before' date. If the date is passed then it means that the food is not at its best. It is safer to use the food before the 'best before' date.

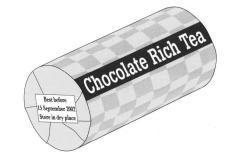

✳ Check date marks in the shop and at home. Use earliest dates first.

✳ Always eat products before the end of their 'use by' date, or cook or freeze for later use.

✳ Check and follow the storage instructions.

✳ Follow any additional instructions, e.g. 'Eat within two days of opening'.

✳ 'If in doubt – throw it out'.

Source: Ministry of Agriculture, Fisheries and Food 1999

Memory Jogger

Write a short paragraph that describes the difference between 'use by', 'sell by' and 'best before'.

Storing food in the refrigerator

Fridge Safety Checklist

✳ Keep the coldest part of the fridge between 0C and 5C (32F and 41F)

✳ Keep a fridge thermometer in the coldest part and check the temperature regularly.

✳ Keep the most perishable foods, like cooked meats, in the coldest part of the fridge.

✳ Return perishable (short shelf life) foods to the fridge or freezer as soon as possible after use.

✳ Wrap or cover all raw or uncooked foods so that they cannot touch or drip on to other foods and contaminate them.

✳ Don't overload the fridge: the cooling air that circulates to keep the fridge cold gets blocked and pockets of warm air form.

✳ Don't put hot food in the fridge: let it cool first.

✳ Don't keep food beyond it's 'use by' date. Check what the label says about refrigeration and shelf life.

✳ Empty any part-used can into a bowl and cover it, otherwise the tin may contaminate the food.

Source: Ministry of Agriculture, Fisheries and Food 1999

Memory Jogger

Use the table on page 111 to help you to answer the questions.

① How can you check to make sure that your fridge is at the correct temperature?

② Where should you keep cooked meats?

③ Why should you wrap or cover raw foods?

④ Draw a simple diagram to show what happens when the fridge is overloaded.

⑤ Mary did not use the whole tin of beans. How should she store the beans that are left in a safe way?

⑥ How cold should the refrigerator be?

What goes where?

10 tips for food shoppers

① If you are not happy with the way food is handled, sold or stored complain to the shop manager or your local environmental health department.

② Always check date codes on food. Do not buy out of date food.

③ If the shop is dirty or has problems with flies or other pests, do not use it and tell the local environmental health department.

④ Do not buy food that looks old, stale or mouldy and make sure the food you get is of the same quality as the food you can see displayed.

⑤ Make sure your food is handled as little as possible and do not accept food which has been handled by anyone with dirty hands or clothes.

⑥ Do not accept ready to eat 'open' food, which has been handled by someone who has also handled raw food, especially raw meat, without thoroughly washing their hands in between.

⑦ Do not accept food served to you by someone who is smoking or eating or has just touched their mouth or hair.

⑧ Only buy cooked meat or cooked meat products, which are kept under refrigeration if the refrigerator has a thermometer make sure it reads 8°C or less.

⑨ Do not buy frozen food, which is soft or defrosting.

⑩ Make sure food packaging is undamaged.

Chartered institute of environmental health

Memory Jogger

Read the 'Ten tips for food shoppers' and answer the questions.

a) What temperature should cooked meat be stored at?

b) What should you do if you are not happy with the way food is being handled in the shop?

c) Make a list of when you should not buy food.

---

4. ENSURING A SAFE ENVIRONMENT

Every year over 125,000 children need hospital treatment from accidents, which happen in the garden. Most of them could have been avoided.

Accidents can happen during times of stress when the normal routine has been changed or when people are in a hurry.

The largest number of accidents happens in the living room/dining room.

Most accidents happen in the late afternoon and early evening, in the summer, during school holidays and at weekends.

The most serious accidents happen in the kitchen and on the stairs.

Those most at risk from a home accident are the 0–4 years age group.

Falls account for the majority of non-fatal accidents.

Every year over 67,000 children experience an accident in the kitchen – 45,000 of these are aged between 0 and 4 years.

54,000 children have accidents on the stairs.

The highest number of deaths is due to fire.

Three children die as a result of a home accident every week.

Source: Home accident surveillance system 1997

Memory Jogger

Use the chart above to help you answer the questions.

Where do the most serious accidents happen?

A   In the garden
B   In the kitchen and on the stairs
C   In the living room and dining room
D   In the kitchen and dining room

When are accidents most likely to happen?

A   In the morning
B   At lunch-time
C   In the late afternoon
D   Before going to bed

The largest number of accidents happen in

A   the garden
B   the kitchen and on the stairs
C   the living room and dining room
D   the kitchen and dining room

The children at greatest risk from home accidents are aged between

A   0–1 years
B   0–2 years
C   0–3 years
D   0–4 years

What time of year are accidents most likely to happen?

A   Spring
B   Summer
C   Autumn
D   Winter

The highest number of deaths are due to

A   Electricity
B   Water
C   Fire
D   Poison

How many children have accidents in the kitchen each year?

A   45000
B   54000
C   67000
D   125000

How many children die each week due to accidents in the home?

A   1
B   2
C   3
D   4

KEY TASKS

Look at the situations described on page 115. Why are these children likely to have accidents? List as many reasons as you can.

Why do children have accidents?

Two children crossing the road between parked cars that they cannot see over. Cars are approaching.

A child playing in poor circumstances.

A child standing on a wobbly stool reaching up to a toy that has been placed on a high cupboard.

A child closing a car door with their fingers around the door framework.

A lost child in a busy shopping area.

A small child behind a table with a hot dish on top of it.

Two older children wrestling with each other.

A child playing with a hammer and pegs and talking to another child behind him/her.

Your answers may have included some of the reasons given below.

✳ Children may not be tall enough to see potential dangers.
✳ Children do not always understand the consequences of their actions.
✳ Children become involved in what they are doing and are not aware of what is happening around them.
✳ They lack experience.
✳ Children are naturally curious but it can lead to danger.
✳ Children like to show off and go beyond their own abilities, especially when there are friends around. Many accidents are caused by horseplay involving pushing, shoving and wrestling.
✳ Accidents are more likely to happen if the child is not supervised.
✳ Some accidents happen because the child is not familiar with the surroundings that he/she is in, e.g. visiting a friend or on holiday.
✳ Poor housing and overcrowded conditions can lead to an increased number of accidents.

Safety in the home

Accidents are the commonest cause of death in children over one year of age. Every year they leave many thousands permanently disabled or disfigured.

The most serious accidents happen in the kitchen and on stairs.

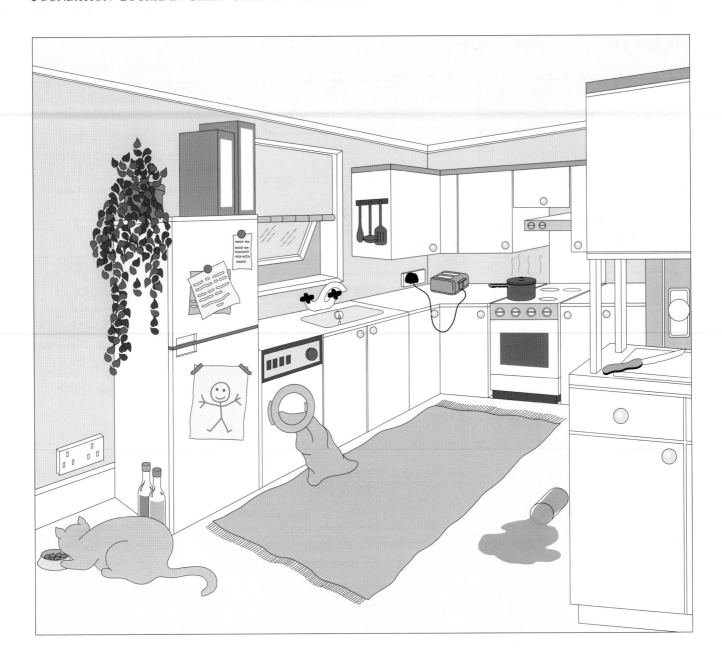

KEY TASKS

✳ Make a list of the potential hazards in the kitchen.

✳ Visit a number of different shops that sell safety equipment for kitchens. Make notes of the different types of equipment and what they are used for.

✳ Design a poster for a parent, which shows how they could make their kitchen a safer place for young children.

What potential hazards can you predict on stairs? List as many as you can.

Toy safety

Toys that are unsafe can still be found on sale in the UK, but they are illegal. When you are choosing or buying toys for children to play with it is very important that you check that they are safe.

 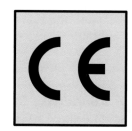 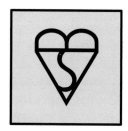

1. European Community (CE) symbol

If you see this marks it tells you that the supplier claims that the toy meets the requirements of the EC Toy Safety Directive. If this symbol is not there it may be that it is being sold as a novelty and is not safe for children to play with.

2. British Toy Manufacturers Association 'Lion Mark'

3. The 'Kite' Mark

Take extra care if you buy toys from car boot sales or jumble sales.

Toys that use batteries

Fit the batteries the right way round, matching at the + and − marks on the battery and the toy.

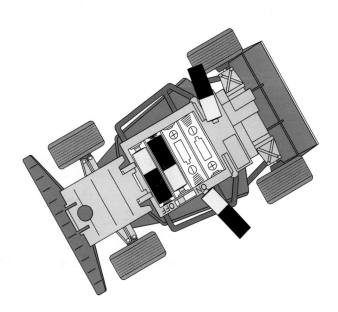

If you need more than one battery, use the same type and always replace a complete set.

Remove old batteries from toys. Never dispose of them in places where they will come into contact with fire.

Store unused batteries in their packaging and away from metal objects, which may cause them to short circuit.

Never try to recharge ordinary batteries either in a battery charger or by applying heat to them.

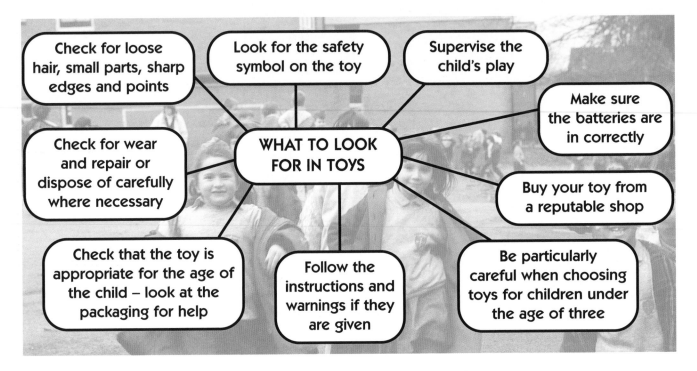

Check for loose hair, small parts, sharp edges and points

Look for the safety symbol on the toy

Supervise the child's play

Make sure the batteries are in correctly

Check for wear and repair or dispose of carefully where necessary

WHAT TO LOOK FOR IN TOYS

Buy your toy from a reputable shop

Check that the toy is appropriate for the age of the child – look at the packaging for help

Follow the instructions and warnings if they are given

Be particularly careful when choosing toys for children under the age of three

5. PROTECTING CHILDREN

Most children live in homes which are loving and caring. However, members or friends of the family abuse some children.

Different types of abuse

* Physical abuse – Non accidental injury (NAI) is when someone deliberately hurts a child
* Sexual abuse
* Emotional abuse
* Neglect

Did you know?

You can cause brain injuries when you toss a young child up in the air.

SIGNS OF ABUSE	
PHYSICAL ABUSE	✳ Bruising which is in the same place on the arms or legs. There may also be bruising in unusual places e.g. under the arm pit, at the back of the knees ✳ Broken bones ✳ Burns and scalds e.g. burns from cigarettes, irons, kettles, bath ✳ Bites and grazes ✳ Internal injuries e.g. head injuries caused by shaking the baby
SEXUAL ABUSE	✳ Itching or pain in the genital area ✳ Withdrawn ✳ Bruises and cuts ✳ Discharge from the penis or vagina
EMOTIONAL ABUSE	✳ Withdrawn ✳ Attention seeking ✳ Easily upset ✳ Tells lies or steals ✳ Low self esteem
NEGLECT	✳ Very thin ✳ Dirty ✳ Tired, hungry, lacks energy ✳ Not well ✳ Often has accidents

What to do if you suspect a child is being abused

In a child care setting

✳ Do not jump to conclusions.
✳ Talk to your work experience supervisor.
✳ The setting will then follow their child protection procedures.

In a family setting

✳ Do not jump to conclusions.
✳ Get advice from the NSPCC (National Society for the Protection of Children).

6. FIRST AID

Anyone working with young children should attend a recognised first aid course. The information in this chapter will give you some basic first aid information.

What is first aid?

First aid is the first help or treatment that is given to a person who has had an accident or is unwell.

What to do if you are on your own

① Find out what has happened.

② Deal with any immediate dangers that may harm you or the person.

③ Keep calm.

④ Ask someone to get help.

⑤ Give first aid.

What to do if your are in a child care setting

① On your first day, find out what the first aid procedures are.

② Follow the procedures.

③ Tell your supervisor what has happened.

KEY TASKS

When you visit a child care setting or during your work experience, find out what the first aid procedures are.

Write the procedures out in a simple list so that you know how to follow them quickly and easily.

Giving first aid when you are on your own

✳ Make sure that the situation is not dangerous for yourself e.g.

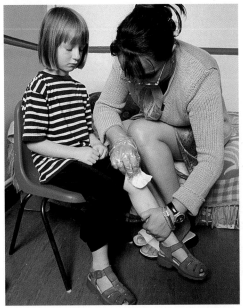

electric wires, fire, chemical spills.

✳ If the child is unconscious, use the ABC procedure see page 121/122.

✳ Ask someone to go for help. It could be another child.

✳ Deal with the most serious injury first.

✳ Reassure the child.

✳ Deal with the minor injuries.

Dial 999 for medical help if the child:

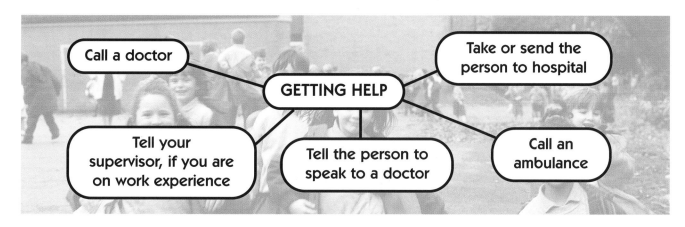

- Call a doctor
- Take or send the person to hospital
- **GETTING HELP**
- Tell your supervisor, if you are on work experience
- Tell the person to speak to a doctor
- Call an ambulance

✳ has no pulse or has stopped breathing

✳ is unconscious or was unconscious immediately after the accident happened

✳ has difficulty breathing

✳ is bleeding badly

✳ has poisoned themselves

✳ has clinical shock, e.g. the child may be allergic to wasp stings or peanuts

✳ has broken a leg or arm

✳ has burnt themselves badly.

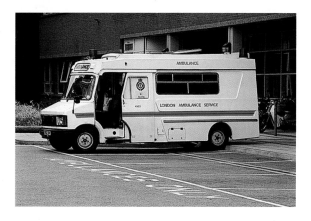

Preventing the spread of infection when giving first aid

✳ Wash your hands before helping the child.

✳ Wear disposable gloves.

✳ If you use materials to clean the wound, wrap them up in the disposable gloves as you take them off.

✳ Put the waste materials into a bag and seal it before putting it into specially marked bag.

✳ Wash your hands when you have finished.

What to do if the child's breathing stops

The ABC procedure for resuscitation

> **A** is for airway
> **B** is for breathing
> **C** is for circulation

Resuscitation for a baby and child

Step 1 – Is the child responding?

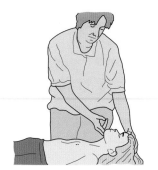

* Check to see if the baby or child responds to you calling their name.
* Tap the bottom of the baby's feet or gently shake the shoulders if the child is older.

Step 2 – Is the airway open and the child breathing?

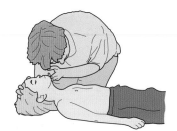

* Open airway and check breathing.
* If it is a baby, put one finger under the baby's chin and gently lift the chin. Check for breathing. If the baby is breathing, cradle the child with their head tilted down.
* If it is a child, place two fingers under the child's chin and gently lift the chin. If the child is breathing, put the child into the recovery position.

Step 3 – Giving artificial ventilation

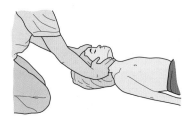

* Make sure that nothing is blocking the airway. Lift the baby's chin and place your mouth over the nose and mouth of the baby. Give five breaths of artificial ventilation.
* If the child is older, only cover the mouth and pinch the child's nose. Give five breaths of artificial ventilation.

Did you know?

A child's pulse beats up to 100 times a minute. An adults pulse beats 60–80 times a minute.

Step 4 – Checking the pulse

✳ Check the baby's pulse in the arm or the child's pulse in the neck.

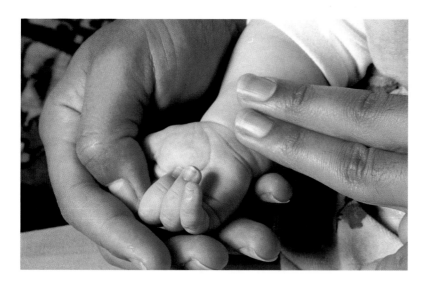

✳ If there is a pulse, continue with the artificial ventilation.
✳ If there is no pulse or if the pulse is less than 60 you will need to give the baby CPR

Step 5 – Starting CPR

Get someone to call an ambulance

✳ **For a baby**
Place two fingers on the lower breastbone. Press down five times. Give a breath of artificial ventilation. Give CPR until the ambulance arrives.

✳ **For a child**
Put the heel of one hand on the child's chest. Press down five times. Give one breath of artificial ventilation. Give CPR until the ambulance arrives.

Burns and scalds

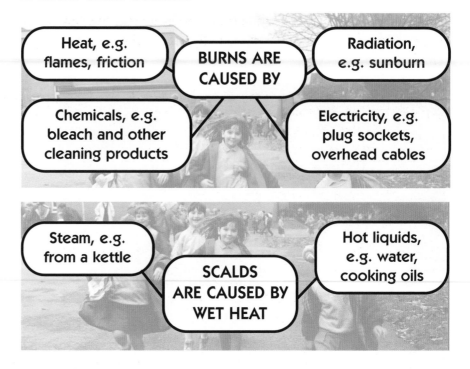

Heat, e.g. flames, friction

BURNS ARE CAUSED BY

Radiation, e.g. sunburn

Chemicals, e.g. bleach and other cleaning products

Electricity, e.g. plug sockets, overhead cables

Steam, e.g. from a kettle

SCALDS ARE CAUSED BY WET HEAT

Hot liquids, e.g. water, cooking oils

Treating minor burns and scalds

DO'S	DON'TS
Get medical help immediately if the child has been badly burned	Do not touch the burn
Soak the burn in cold water or put the burn under slow running water for at least ten minutes	Do not burst any blisters that appear on the skin
Carefully take off any jewellery before the area begins to swell	Do not remove clothing if it is sticking to the burn. It can cause more damage
Cover the burn with a clean, sterile dressing	Do not use a fluffy dressing or a plaster
If a small area has been burned and you are concerned about it, take the child to the Health Centre	Do not use any creams, fat or ointments on the burn

KEY TASKS

Steven left a hot cup of coffee on the low table in the living room. His three year-old daughter knocked the table and the coffee spilt over her arm.

① Was this a burn or a scald?

② What should Steven do?

③ How could Steven have prevented this accident from happening?

Choking

A child chokes when something blocks their airway. Swallowing a large piece of food or an object usually causes choking in young children.

DO'S
Look inside the child's mouth. If you can see what is causing the child to choke and it will come out easily, hook it out with your finger. If it is stuck, leave it alone.
If you cannot remove the object, put the child face down across your knees. The child's head should be lower than his/her chest.
Slap the child four or five times between his/her shoulder blades.
Turn the child over and look to see if it is possible to remove the object.
Make sure the child is breathing.
If the child is not breathing, start the resuscitation procedure.
Get medical help immediately.

DONT'S
Never hold a baby or child upside down by the ankles and slap their back. You could break their neck.

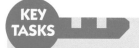

Linda is five years old and she has swallowed a marble. What should you do?

Drowning

① Dial 999 immediately.

② Remove the child from the water, keeping the head as still as possible.

③ Check ABC.

④ If the child is not breathing, begin rescue breathing. Do not bend the child's neck back if you think the child has hurt its neck or is unconscious.

⑤ When the child starts to breath again, treat for shock.

⑥ If the child is not breathing carrying on the rescue breathing.

⑦ Cover the child with warm clothing or blankets.

⑧ Talk to the child and reassure them while you wait on medical help coming.

Cuts and bleeding

If you help a child who has a cut or is bleeding, always wear disposable gloves to stop cross infection.

Minor cuts and grazes

DO'S	DON'TS
Talk to the child and reassure them.	
Sit or lie them down.	
Clean the area with cold water.	Do not try to take out pieces of grit.
Put on a dressing if necessary.	Do not use plasters that could cause an allergy. Do not use ointments or creams.
Record the incident in the Accident Report Book.	
Make sure the parent/carer knows about the incident.	

Severe bleeding

1. Dial 999 immediately.
2. Wear disposable gloves.
3. Talk to the child and reassure them.
4. Put pressure on the bleeding, e.g. use a clean tea towel. Do not use fluffy materials.
5. Lift the cut if possible, e.g. if it is on an arm or leg.
6. Put on a sterile dressing.
7. If the blood soaks through, do not take the dressing off. Put a new dressing on top.
8. Keep the child warm.
9. Do not give the child anything to eat or drink.
10. Get in touch with the parent/carer.

TEST YOURSELF

① Personal hygiene is very important. Describe **four** ways of having good personal hygiene.

② How is infection spread? Give **three** examples.

③ Fill in the missing words.

How to stop infection spreading

Children can be _____ against infectious disease.

Toys and play equipment should be _____

It is important to _____ your hands after you have used the toilet.

You should always wear _____ when changing children's nappies.

If a person has an infectious disease they may be put into an _____ ward.

isolation	immunised	wash	disinfectant	disposable gloves

④ What should the coldest part of the refrigerator be kept at?

⑤ Where should you store cooked meats?

⑥ Most accidents happen in the home. Give **five** ways of preventing accidents in the kitchen.

⑦ Why do children have accidents? Give **three** reasons.

⑧ How do you know a toy is safe?

⑨ What does ABC mean in first aid?

⑩ What is the difference between a scald and a burn?

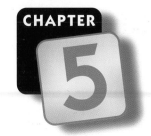
Looking After Children

* The basic needs of children
* Caring for children

1. THE BASIC NEEDS OF CHILDREN

We all have needs. Some of these needs are essential in order to grow and develop.

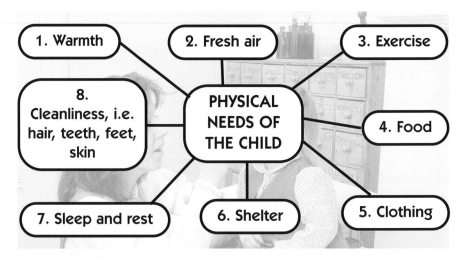

| 1. Warmth | 2. Fresh air | 3. Exercise |

| 8. Cleanliness, i.e. hair, teeth, feet, skin | PHYSICAL NEEDS OF THE CHILD | 4. Food |

| 7. Sleep and rest | 6. Shelter | 5. Clothing |

WHAT YOUNG CHILDREN NEED	
At birth	Warmth and quiet Cleanliness Firm but gentle handling and head supported Being talked to when they are awake
One month	Regular daily routine Feeding altered to the child's needs and the needs of the mother Talked to regularly
Three months	Chance to stretch and wriggle Cuddled and talked to A chance to splash and play in the bath

WHAT YOUNG CHILDREN NEED cont.

Six months	Freedom to kick and roll about safely
	Opportunities to sit up but be supported
	Finger rhymes with adult
	Simple toys, e.g. rattle, rings to bite, wooden cubes, large beads
Nine months	Safe place to crawl and play
	A variety of toys, e.g. small bricks, balls, dolls
	Clothes that let the child crawl and roll about in
	Time to play in the bath
	Time with adults
	Simple nursery rhymes, stories, songs
	Appropriate diet
	Daily routine changed to allow for more activity
One year	Opportunities to stand, crawl and try to walk safely
	Protection from accidents in the home
	Encouragement from adults
	Music, songs, books
	Suitable clothes
	Sufficient sleep and a balanced diet
2 years	Simple stories, finger play and songs
	Simple games with adults
	Sand, water, bricks, dolls, boxes, push and pull toys
	Comfort when frightened, especially at night
	Firmness when necessary
3 years	Opportunities to play with other children
	Praise and encouragement
	As much independence as possible
	Dress up clothes, painting, drawing, modelling, building
	Sand and water play
	Stories, books, songs
4 years	Opportunities for physical and imaginative play in a safe environment
	Large play material for building
	More advanced books, songs
5 years	Play materials similar to the four year-old
	Support from parent when child starts school
6 and 7 years	Patience from parents and teachers
	Firm control over daily routine
	Praise and encouragement
	Sufficient rest and sleep
	Protection against over tiredness

Adapted from Lee, C. The growth and development of children

CARING FOR A CHILD'S PHYSICAL NEEDS

1. Warmth

Our normal body temperature is between 36–37.5°C. We can get hotter or colder depending on what we are doing and what the outside temperature is. Very young babies should be kept in a room temperature of between 16 and 20°C.

If we become very cold we will suffer from hypothermia. If we get too hot, we become dehydrated and can develop a heat rash. Sudden Infant Death Syndrome (SIDS) has been linked to babies becoming too hot.

2. Fresh air

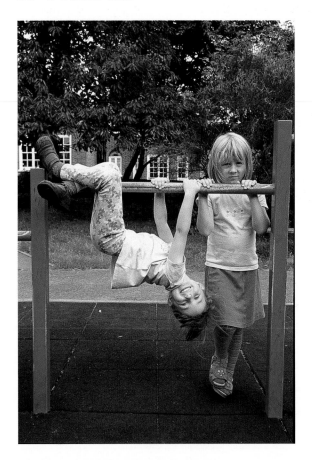

All children should spend some time outside during the day. They should wear clothes which are appropriate for the weather, e.g. warm clothes, waterproof clothing, or light clothes which keep them cool but protect them from the sun.

How do children benefit from being in the fresh air?

✸ Fresh air can give children energy.

✸ It can improve their appetite.

✸ The sunlight can kill bacteria and can encourage the skin to produce Vitamin D.

✸ It helps them sleep at night.

✸ They will look healthy.

Some children are allergic to grass cuttings or rape seed (these are bright yellow flowers which are grown by farmers and flower in April/May and have a very strong smell).

The air can be polluted due to smoke from factories and carbon monoxide from cars. Lead-free petrol can be bought. This helps to reduce the high levels of lead in the air, which can cause brain damage in young children. Air pollution can also cause breathing problems, e.g. asthma.

3. Exercise

Years ago, children spent most of their spare time playing outside. Today children spend their free time indoors watching television, playing on the computer or sitting on the sofa.

Children should be active for at least an hour every day, e.g. playing football, walking to school, playing basketball, cycling. Regular exercise:

✸ improves balance

✸ strengthens muscles

✸ makes the heart and lungs more efficient

✸ improves physical and mental health.

Did you know?

Active children do better in class but 33% of boys and 38% of girls aged two to seven are not meeting the recommended daily activity levels.

4. Food

We all need a healthy balanced diet to grow and develop. To find out more about the importance of a healthy diet, read Chapter 4 in this book.

5. Clothing

Choosing footwear

Did you know?

Our feet will carry us the equivalent of five times round the earth in an average lifetime.

✸ A baby's foot is not a smaller version of an adult's foot. It is shorter, wider and tapers towards the heel. When the baby is born, the foot is very soft and can be damaged very easily.

✸ The baby's foot grows very quickly in the first year.

✳ When the child first begins to walk, shoes are not necessary indoors. Allowing the child to go barefoot or to wear just socks helps the foot to grow normally.

✳ When the baby is outside, the feet should be protected in lightweight shoes made of natural materials.

✳ A child does not need shoes until it is walking without help.

✳ Always go to a shoe shop, which will measure the child's feet.

✳ As the child grows, it may be necessary to change shoes every few months to allow room for the feet to grow.

✳ Children should not wear shoes that have been worn by other children. The shoe will have changed shape and will not fit the child.

Memory Jogger

How many words can you find?

**Muscle   Constipation   Co-ordination
Sleep   Digestion   Central nervous system
Body fat   Lungs**

C	O	O	R	D	I	N	A	T	I	O	N
E	X	L	U	N	G	S	N	L	F	M	M
N	P	O	W	C	U	Y	D	G	G	H	U
T	S	T	E	O	P	S	G	F	Q	J	S
R	L	A	V	B	W	T	I	C	Z	C	C
A	E	R	T	Z	O	E	P	B	I	K	L
L	E	P	R	Q	I	M	P	B	T	L	E
N	P	N	O	I	T	S	E	G	I	D	R
N	O	I	T	A	P	I	T	S	N	O	C

Use the words above to fill in the missing spaces.
Exercise strengthens the _____ in the body. It can help to encourage _____ as the body needs to relax afterwards. It prevents the build up of _____ _____ as exercise increases the number of kilojoules/calories used. It improves _____ by training the _____ _____ _____ through repetition and skill. Exercise helps the development of the _____ It can also improve the digestion of food and helps prevent _____

Different types of footwear for children

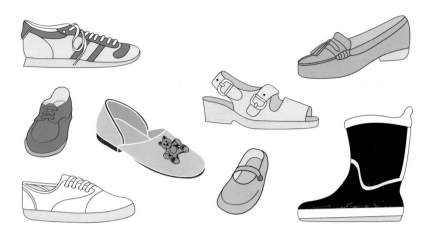

Choosing shoes for children

Source: www.feetforlife.org/kidshoe.htm

Always have both feet measured for length and width by a trained fitter.

Shoes should be held on the foot with laces, straps or Velcro. It is best to avoid slip on shoes.

Flat shoes are best for children.

The shoe should fit the natural shape of the foot especially round the toes.

CHOOSING SHOES FOR CHILDREN

Choose shoes with leather uppers. Nylon, plastic and rubber can cause athlete's foot and toenail problems.

The toe of the shoe should let the toes move freely and not be squashed. There should be about 18 mm growing room between the end of the longest toe and the end of the shoe.

Shoes should fit comfortably around the heel and not be too loose or too tight.

Fashion shoes are good for special occasions but not for everyday wear.

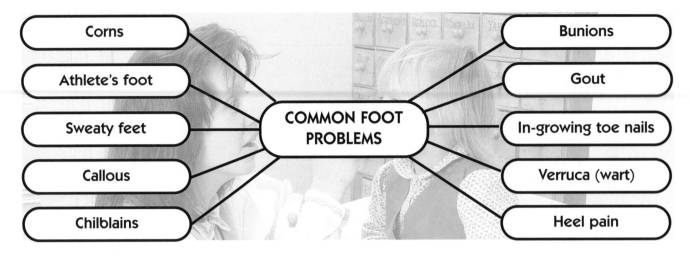

COMMON FOOT PROBLEMS

- Corns
- Athlete's foot
- Sweaty feet
- Callous
- Chilblains
- Bunions
- Gout
- In-growing toe nails
- Verruca (wart)
- Heel pain

Choosing clothes for babies

The first set of clothes that are bought for the baby has traditionally been called the layette . A new parent often receives gifts of clothes before or after the baby is born. It is important to know what is suitable for babies at different stages in their development.

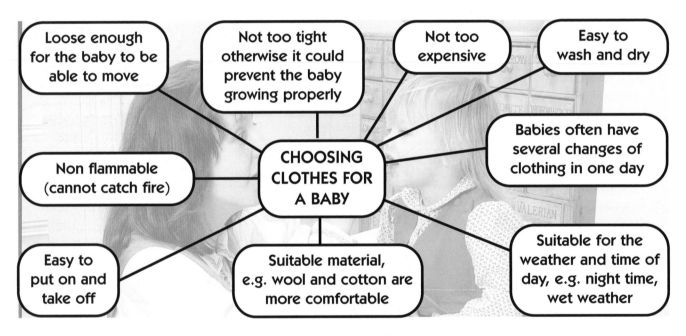

CHOOSING CLOTHES FOR A BABY

- Loose enough for the baby to be able to move
- Not too tight otherwise it could prevent the baby growing properly
- Not too expensive
- Easy to wash and dry
- Babies often have several changes of clothing in one day
- Non flammable (cannot catch fire)
- Easy to put on and take off
- Suitable material, e.g. wool and cotton are more comfortable
- Suitable for the weather and time of day, e.g. night time, wet weather

A baby's wardrobe

✳ Nappies (either disposable or Terry nappies)
✳ Waterproof pants to wear over the nappy. These help to keep the baby's clothes and bedding dry.
✳ Vest
✳ Baby grows and stretch suits – these are easy to wash and cover the baby from 'top to toe'
✳ Socks, hat, mittens
✳ Cardigans
✳ Bibs
✳ All in one suit for the buggy

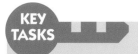

KEY TASKS

Visit a shop that sells baby clothes. Using the list above as a guide, find out how much it would cost to buy clothes for a new baby.

Choosing clothes for children

Young children love to play and as a result they often get dirty. Children grow very quickly. Choosing the right clothes for the right situation is very important.

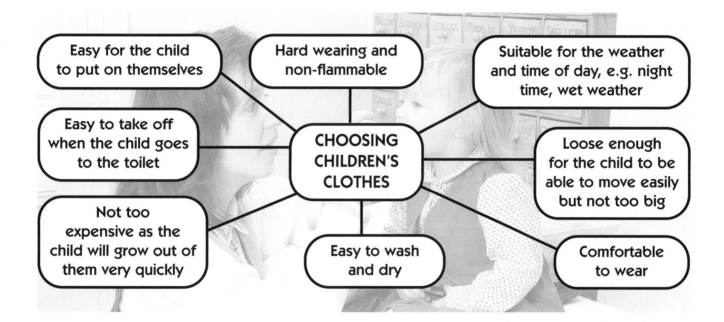

- Easy for the child to put on themselves
- Hard wearing and non-flammable
- Suitable for the weather and time of day, e.g. night time, wet weather
- Easy to take off when the child goes to the toilet
- **CHOOSING CHILDREN'S CLOTHES**
- Loose enough for the child to be able to move easily but not too big
- Not too expensive as the child will grow out of them very quickly
- Easy to wash and dry
- Comfortable to wear

Clothes for night time

Baby All in one pyjamas keep the baby warm, especially when they kick off the covers.

Older children Pyjamas are easy to take off if the child needs to go to the toilet during the night.

A night shirt is good during the summer as it is cooler to wear but not so warm for the winter. A dressing gown keeps the child warm when they are getting ready for bed.

Clothes for the day time

Baby During the day the baby needs clothes suitable for the weather, comfortable and allows them to move freely.

Older children Playsuits and dungarees are good for children who are crawling. It helps to hold their nappy in place but keeps them warm. However, dungarees should not be worn when the child is being toilet trained as they are difficult to get off quickly. Playing in dresses and skirts can be very restrictive.

T-shirts, cotton jumpers, track suits, trousers, shorts.

Outdoors   Anoraks or jackets with hood, hat, scarf and gloves will keep the child warm and dry.

A sun hat with a broad rim will protect the child from burning.

A one-piece waterproof suit is useful for younger children.

KEY TASKS

You are working as a mother's help for a three year old child and a six month old baby. It is a warm summer's day but rain is forecast. You are going with the parent and the children on a picnic to the seaside.

What clothes should the children wear to travel to the seaside?

What clothes do you need to take with you?

6. A home

Many children have a home, which is clean and is a safe and protected environment.

Home should be where the child can:

✳ keep its own toys and possessions
✳ receive praise and encouragement from an adult
✳ have space to play on their own or with others
✳ take part in day to day routines, e.g. laying the table.

Poor housing can lead to health problems.

Poor ventilation encourages house mites

Fungal spores from dampness

Asthma and other breathing difficulties and long term illnesses

Chemicals from gas appliances

Lead poisoning

Breathing problems

Carbon monoxide poisoning

Death

7. Sleep and rest

Newborn babies are asleep most of the time. They only wake up when they are hungry. A range of different equipment can be bought for the baby to sleep in.

Why are rest and sleep important?
✳ Children need to rest and sleep to stay healthy.
✳ The body has time to relax.
✳ Children who have enough sleep are less likely to be ill.
✳ Children who are tired are often bad-tempered and 'do not know what to do with themselves'.

Sleep patterns

On average:

Baby	16 hours a day
1 year old	14 hours a day
Over 1 year of age	One nap per day
4 year old	12 hours
Over 5 years of age	Most children outgrow the need for a nap during the day
8 year old	9 hours

A bedtime routine can help the child get to sleep each night. It gives the child a chance to relax after a busy day and it gives the adult the chance to spend some time with the child.

Bedtime routine

✳ Bath
✳ Teeth brushing
✳ Bedtime story

8. Cleanliness

All children enjoy getting dirty but after the fun, children should wash to prevent infection. The adult must make sure that the child's hair, skin, teeth and feet and cared for.

Caring for a child's skin

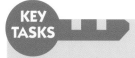

KEY TASKS

Design a poster, which explains how to care for the skin.

Our skin is the first part of our body that comes into contact with the environment. It is very important that we care for it and protect it.

Caring for a child's hair

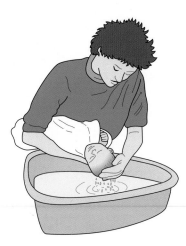

Baby

* Be very gentle.
* Avoid putting pressure on the soft spot on the top of the baby's head.
* Make sure there are no tangles in the hair before washing it.
* Only do it when you have to. It does not have to be done every day.
* Use a baby or very mild shampoo.
* It is often better to wash the baby's hair while giving them their bath.
* Support the baby so that they are on their back with their head facing the ceiling.
* Check that the water is not too hot.

Pre-school child

* Many young children do not like having their hair washed. However, it is important to teach children that keeping their hair clean is important.
* Keep the water out of their eyes by using goggles or a visor.
* Tell the child what you are going to do before you do it.
* Avoid pouring large amounts of water over the child's head. Use your hands to rinse a little bit at a time.
* Encourage the child to lean back over the sink or bath. This can prevent water going onto the face.
* Use a gentle shampoo. Do not use too much.
* Encourage the child to join in e.g. they can lather their own head.

✳ Do not wash the child's hair too often. Once or twice a week is enough.

School-aged child

As children get older they start to have an opinion of how they want to wear their hair. This is a good time to teach them how to care for their own hair, e.g. combing and brushing their hair, detangling and using clean brushes and combs.

Caring for children's teeth

Children have two sets of teeth in their lifetime. They will have 20 milk teeth and 32 permanent teeth.

Poor diet or use of certain types of medication during pregnancy can cause the baby's teeth and permanent teeth to be discoloured, damaged or even misshapen. Primary teeth will fall out, but they can get cavities and may need to be treated. If the primary teeth fall out too quickly, it can cause problems when the permanent teeth come in.

Baby

The baby's first tooth will appear at about six months old. It is usually the lower incisor. Sometimes teething can begin as early as three to four months. Babies' teeth can get plaque so it is important to wipe them gently.

Older children

> **Did you know?**
>
> By the sixth week of pregnancy, the baby's teeth are already starting to form.

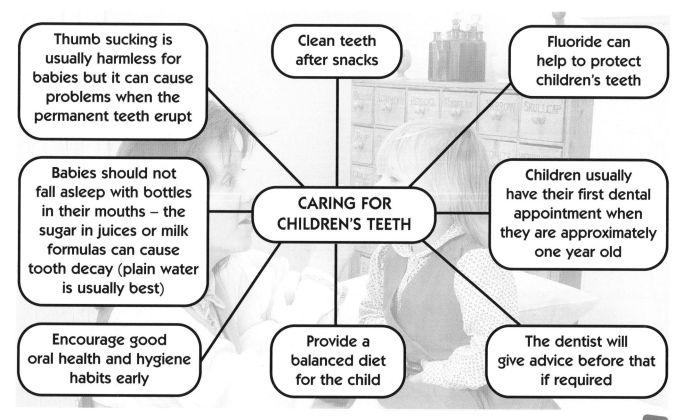

Thumb sucking is usually harmless for babies but it can cause problems when the permanent teeth erupt

Clean teeth after snacks

Fluoride can help to protect children's teeth

Babies should not fall asleep with bottles in their mouths – the sugar in juices or milk formulas can cause tooth decay (plain water is usually best)

CARING FOR CHILDREN'S TEETH

Children usually have their first dental appointment when they are approximately one year old

Encourage good oral health and hygiene habits early

Provide a balanced diet for the child

The dentist will give advice before that if required

Brushing teeth

Children can learn how to brush their own teeth, but they will need help.

✳ When they clean the lower teeth they should brush up and away from the gums. When they clean the upper teeth they should brush down and away from the gums.

✳ The back teeth are the most difficult teeth to clean. Young children will need help to clean their back teeth.

Taking a child to the dentist for the first time

✳ Let the child watch you at home when you are cleaning and checking your teeth.

✳ Read books to the child about the topic.

✳ Take the child to the dentist when you go.

✳ Explain that a dentist will look at their teeth to see if everything is OK.

✳ Talk to the dentist about how to keep children's teeth clean and healthy.

KEY TASKS

When you go to the dentist ask them how they help young children when they visit the dentist.

Other basic needs

A child does not just have physical needs. The child also needs to be safe, feel loved and valued.

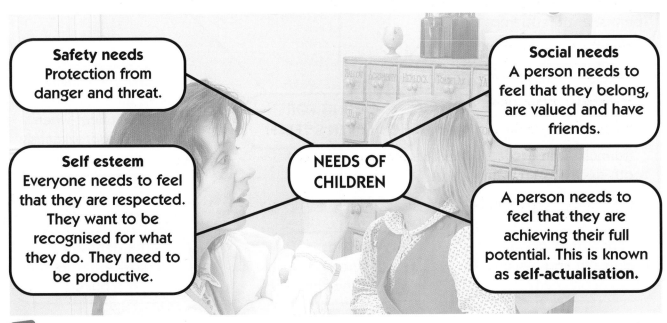

Safety needs
Protection from danger and threat.

Social needs
A person needs to feel that they belong, are valued and have friends.

Self esteem
Everyone needs to feel that they are respected. They want to be recognised for what they do. They need to be productive.

NEEDS OF CHILDREN

A person needs to feel that they are achieving their full potential. This is known as **self-actualisation**.

TEST YOURSELF

① List the eight basic needs of a child.

② What is our normal body temperature?

③ Why is fresh air important for a young child? Give three reasons.

④ Why does a baby's foot damage very easily?

⑤ When should a parent buy a child's first pair of shoes?

⑥ How many milk teeth does a child have?

10   15   20   25   (Circle the correct answer)

How many permanent teeth does a child have?

26   28   30   32   (Circle the correct answer)

⑦

P	R	O	T	E	C	T	I	O	N
V	G	T	G	P	N	S	J	N	N
I	E	B	C	D	Q	V	O	Q	O
T	R	O	Z	F	G	I	N	P	I
A	M	W	A	S	T	E	S	B	T
M	S	P	L	A	A	M	I	F	E
I	T	R	S	W	E	A	T	K	R
N	L	N	G	H	K	X	C	L	C
S	S	T	C	U	D	O	R	P	S

Find the functions of the skin in the word search.

Secretion   Germs   Waste products   Sweat

Sensation   Protection   Vitamin D

⑧ What clothes would a parent need to buy for a new baby?

⑨ Poor housing can cause different health problems. Give **four** examples.

⑩ How much sleep should a four year-old child get each day?

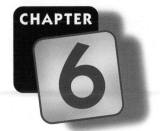
Play and Practical Activities

✳ How play helps a child to learn and develop
✳ Different types of play
✳ What the adult does when the child is playing

1. HOW PLAY HELPS A CHILD TO LEARN AND DEVELOP

Why play?

✳ Play is fun.
✳ Play is an exciting way to learn new skills in a safe and secure environment.
✳ Play helps children get to know other people.
✳ Play can help young children find out more about the environment in which they live.

KEY TASKS

Think back to your own childhood.

a) What games did you play?

b) Who did you play with?

c) What do you think you learned?

d) Complete the table on page 143. When you have finished, compare your answers with a friend.

Play is one way in which children can begin to understand and learn about different experiences.

Children learn through play because they are:

✳ watching (observing) other children and adults
✳ listening to the sounds that they hear

GAMES YOU PLAYED WHEN YOU WERE YOUNG	HOW MANY PLAYED THE GAME WITH YOU?	WHAT DID YOU PLAY WITH?	WHAT DID YOU LEARN WHEN YOU WERE PLAYING?
Example: Houses	Usually I played with my sister	I played underneath the table with dolls, teacups, magazines.	I learned how to share my toys with my sister. I also learned how to look after my dolls. I copied my parents and what they did.

✳ touching different materials, textures
✳ tasting
✳ smelling

How can play help children's learning?

What is this?

What does it smell of?

What does it taste like?

What does it do?

Does it taste nice?

Do I need to follow any rules?

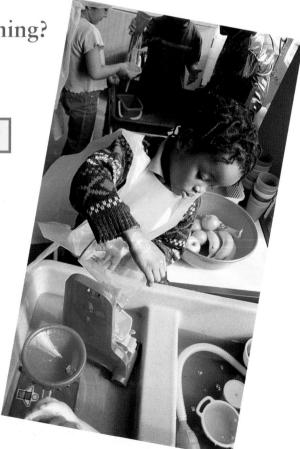

HOW PLAY CAN HELP A CHILD'S LEARNING

PHYSICAL DEVELOPMENT
* Gross motor skills can be practised – they can be repeated as often as necessary
* Improve fine manipulative skills
* Improve muscle tone

INTELLECTUAL DEVELOPMENT
* Discover and learn new concepts (ideas)
* Helps develop memory
* Opportunity to experiment, create and invent in a safe environment
* Develops concentration
* Interesting and stimulating way to learn

LANGUAGE DEVELOPMENT
* Learn new words
* Introduce children to reading
* Encourage listening skills
* Helps to develop sentence structure
* Encourage conversation between people
* Talk about new ideas, exciting events (this shows what the child understands)

SOCIAL DEVELOPMENT
* Co-operate with other people
* Take turns
* Follow rules
* Find out how other people behave
* Opportunity to pretend to be someone else, i.e role play
* Learn to share
* Gain friends
* Understand how to care for others
* Develops independence

EMOTIONAL DEVELOPMENT
* Fun and enjoyable
* Opportunity to express feelings in a safe environment, e.g. anger, bereavement
* Have a sense of control
* Develop positive self esteem and confidence
* Provides a 'way to escape' from the pressures of reality
* Satisfying and relaxing

Memory Jogger

Physical	Listen	Words	Age
Concepts	Stage	Memory	Social
Concentration	Events	Discover	Five

Use the words in the box above to help you to answer fill in the missing spaces.

There are .... main areas of development. Play can help children's ....development by improving their fine manipulative and gross motor skills. When children play together they take ...., learn rules and gain new friends. This promotes their .... development. A child's intellectual development is improved through play because it helps them to .... and learn new .... It can improve their .... and .... A child's language development is also improved because it helps them to .... , learn new .... and talk about exciting .... Play can encourage learning if the activities are appropriate to the child's .... and .... of development.

Choosing play equipment for children

When you are choosing toys and other play equipment for young children to use it is important to consider a number of different factors.

Suitability

The toy or equipment must be suitable for the age of the child and the stage of development that they are at. It is also important to take account of any special needs that the child may have.

Learning value

The toy should allow the child to use his or her imagination and let them experiment. Children become bored if the toy has limited uses.

Durability

Always make sure that the toy is strong enough to withstand a lot of usage.

Safety

The toy must comply with the British safety regulations. A toy that is safe enough for an older child to use may not be safe for a young child.

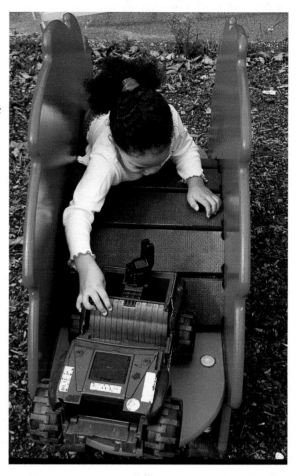

Choosing toys for very young children

Babies need to be able to see and touch things. They like to watch and play with objects that move, have bright colours and make different sounds.

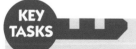

KEY TASKS

Make a mobile for a young baby. It could hang from the ceiling or be attached to a cot or buggy. Think carefully about the shapes and colours that you are going to use.

What do children like to play with?

1 TO 6 MONTHS
* Rattle
* Small blocks
* Teething rings
* Bath toys
* Mobiles
* Pram toys

6 TO 12 MONTHS
* Cubes and beakers
* String of large beads
* Wooden spoons
* Pots and pans
* Soft dolls
* Soft books

12 TO 18 MONTHS
* Cuddly toys
* Hammer and pegs
* Wooden train
* Bath toys
* Boxes, tins, cartons
* Toys to push and pull

18 MONTHS TO 2 YEARS
* Posting box
* Screw toys
* Wooden rings to fit on sticks
* Teddy bear, soft dolls
* Toys to ride on
* Balls
* Dressing up clothes

2 TO 3 YEARS
* Picture books
* Dressing up clothes
* Dolls
* Water and things to pour, tip, fill
* Sand, sieves, spades
* Paints
* Dough, clay
* Balls
* Simple puzzles
* Bricks, Duplo
* Toys to ride on

3 TO 4 YEARS
* Scissors
* Different sizes and shapes of paper
* Jigsaws
* Matching games
* Farm sets, garage, train sets
* Toys that fit together
* Books
* Home area

4 TO 5 YEARS
* Woodwork tools
* Garden tools
* Puppets
* Painting and drawing materials
* Materials to make models, e.g. cereal packets, kitchen rolls
* More complex table top games

5 TO 6 YEARS
* Construction and building sets with smaller pieces
* Writing materials
* Footballs, skipping ropes, scooters
* Table top games
* More complex jigsaws
* Musical instruments

6 TO 7 YEARS
* Needles and thread for sewing
* Bicycle
* Roller blades
* Computer

7 TO 8 YEARS
* Kites
* Fiction and non fiction books

8 TO 12 YEARS
* Model sets
* Chess, draughts
* Tool kits
* Computers
* Electronic games
* Science kits
* Sports equipment

2. DIFFERENT TYPES OF PLAY

There is a range of different types of play that a child can get involved in.

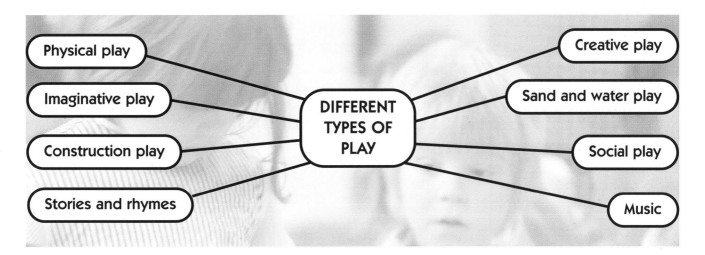

- Physical play
- Imaginative play
- Construction play
- Stories and rhymes

DIFFERENT TYPES OF PLAY

- Creative play
- Sand and water play
- Social play
- Music

Physical play

Physical play is when a child is moving, jumping, running, throwing a ball etc. Children develop different skills when they take part in physical play.

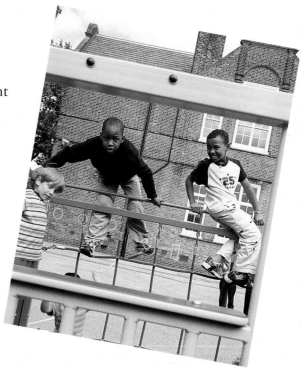

run	skip	hop	walk	jump
roll	balance	stretch	crawl	hide
swing	turn	twist	listen	stamp
pull	shake	hit	push	shoot
reach	kneel	lie	stand	float
whirl	tip toe	gallop	slide	clap

What does a child learn from outdoor physical play?

Sharing the use of equipment
Control of body
Exploring movement in space
Steering, turning
Experiencing speed
Investigating mini beasts, the soil, growing, etc
Hand and eye co-ordination
Caring for plants and animals
Enjoy nature

Confidence
Balance
Self esteem
Recognise objects from different angles
Self control
Learn about safety rules
Test and develop skills
Test courage
Put weight onto different parts of the body
Co-operation
Aware of needs of others
Role play
Language
Sharing equipment

Working with large equipment
Lifting, placing, balancing
Problem solving
Co-operation
Negotiation
Throwing
Skipping
Rolling
Following instructions

KEY TASKS

Visit a local play area and complete the following tasks.

✳ Draw a plan of the play area and name the equipment that is available.

✳ Choose **two** pieces of equipment. What do they encourage the children to do?

✳ What age range do you think could use the equipment safely? Make a note of the age of the children who are playing in the area, if possible.

✳ Make a list of the potential hazards that you can see in the play area.

✳ Describe how the safety of the children has been taken into consideration.

✳ What do you think of the play area?

Safety during physical play

It is essential that the adult makes sure that the area is safe for the children to play in.

Before

* Look to see if any of the equipment is broken or needing repaired. If it is, remove it.
* Look for peeling paint, nails that are sticking out, sharp edges and splinters.
* Check that safety gates are closed.
* Is there enough space between pieces of equipment to move safely?
* Make sure there is no broken glass, dog faeces or other dangerous objects in the play area.
* Check that the safety mats are in place and in good working order.
* Make sure that there are no poisonous berries in the play area.

During play

* Watch the children at all times.
* Help them if they need it but leave them on their own as much as possible to encourage independence and build up their confidence.
* Make sure that there are not too many children using one toy.

After play

* Check the equipment to make sure that nothing has broken or become loose during play.

The role of the adult in physical play

* Provide equipment and activities that are appropriate for the age of the child and their stage of development.
* Praise and encourage the child especially when they are testing their own limits of ability, e.g. when they are standing on the highest point of the climbing frame.
* Make sure the children are safe.

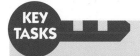

KEY TASKS

Find as many potential hazards as you can in the park picture below.

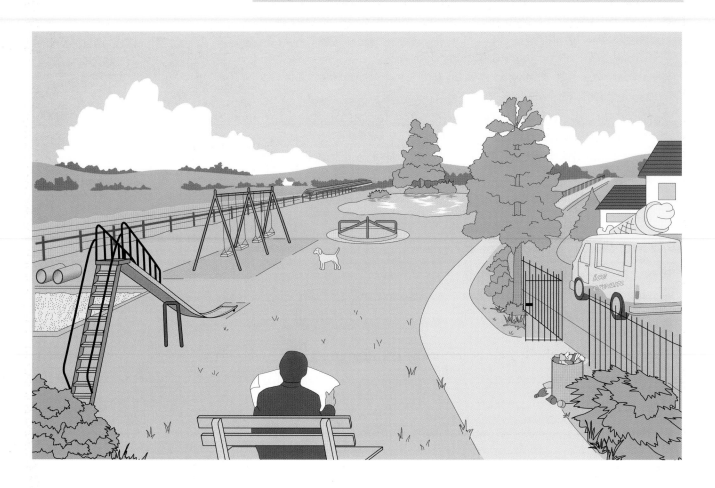

Memory Jogger

How many words can you find?

Self-confidence   Sharing   Digestion   Infection   Circulation   Appetite
Curiosity   Risk   Physical skills   Tension   Vocabulary   Listening
Collaborating   Turn taking   Challenge

S	E	L	F	C	O	N	F	I	D	E	N	C	E	Y
H	L	I	S	T	E	N	I	N	G	Q	E	H	R	T
A	U	I	O	P	S	D	F	F	C	V	G	A	H	J
R	K	L	Z	X	C	V	B	E	N	O	M	L	H	L
I	I	Q	W	E	R	T	Y	C	U	C	A	L	I	O
N	P	S	A	S	D	F	G	T	H	A	P	E	J	K
G	L	Z	K	X	C	V	B	I	N	B	P	N	M	Q
D	W	E	R	U	I	O	P	O	P	U	E	G	A	S
I	D	F	G	H	J	K	L	N	F	L	T	E	G	H
E	H	J	K	I	T	R	E	D	G	R	T	H	U	K
S	C	U	R	I	O	S	I	T	Y	Y	E	B	G	T
T	U	R	N	T	A	K	I	N	G	T	R	E	W	C
I	B	G	N	I	T	A	R	O	B	A	L	L	O	C
O	P	H	Y	S	I	C	A	L	S	K	I	L	L	S
N	O	I	T	A	L	U	C	R	I	C	N	B	G	T

Complete the table below, using the words in the search word. The first one has been done for you.

PHYSICAL	INTELLECTUAL	LANGUAGE	EMOTIONAL	SOCIAL
			Self confidence	

151

Creative Play

Creative play is when a child is able to show their own ideas and feelings by drawing, making models, using different materials and painting. It gives children the chance to communicate without having to talk.

Creative play allows children to use their imagination. The role of the adult is to provide different equipment and materials and allow the children to create their own piece of work.

What does a child learn from creative play?

Intellectual development
Problem solving skills
Finding the right materials and putting them back when finished
Sorting, matching, counting, measuring
Listening and following instructions
Watching, copying others

Language development
Talking about what they have done
Communicate thoughts and feelings through painting and drawing

Social and Emotional development
Fun
Frustration
Helping others
Working through a challenge
Sense of achievement
Satisfaction in completing the task

Physical development
Developing hand and eye co-ordination
Fine manipulative skills
Developing control over the materials

KEY TASKS

Make a file of different creative activities that you could use with children of different ages. The first page could show the different types of paper that are available to use for creative play (see page 155).

Different activities and equipment that can promote creative play

Painting and drawing

Painting and drawing can promote the all round development of a young child.

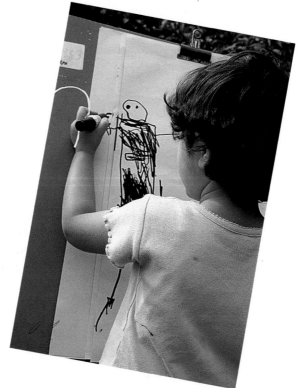

> **Physical**
> Holding the brush helps in the development of fine motor skill
> Control
> Hand and eye co-ordination is required

> **Intellectual**
> The child becomes more aware of shape, colour, texture, line
> Problem solving
> Increased concentration

> **PAINTING AND DRAWING**

> **Emotional**
> Relaxing, fun
> Use painting as a means of expressing feelings, e.g. anger, fear, sadness

> **Social**
> Sharing materials
> Taking turns
> Paint social situations

> **Language**
> Important form of communication
> Vocabulary is increased and understood
> Ability to follow instructions and show understanding

What a child has to learn in order to paint and draw successfully

It is important to know what skills the child needs to have so that the equipment and activities provided for the child are appropriate.

Painting

* How to hold a brush
* Dipping it into the pot
* Taking off excess paint
* Applying the paint to the paper
* Using different brushes
* Choosing suitable paints
* Using paper of different weights
* Preparing paints
* Cleaning and storing equipment

Glueing

* Spreading glue
* Positioning materials
* Choosing appropriate glues for what they want to do
* Controlling the quantity of glue
* Storing and cleaning equipment

Cutting

* Holding scissors correctly. Children who are left-handed should have access to left-handed scissors.
* Mastering the biting action
* Snipping, fringing, strips
* Following a line and curve
* Cutting shapes and different materials
* Carrying scissors safely
* Storing scissors

Tearing

* Controlled tearing
* Tearing along a line or shape
* Tearing different textures
* Tearing holes

Crayons/chalks

* Holding crayons
* Experiencing filling in and rubbing
* Using different edges
* Exploring lines, colour and texture

DIFFERENT TYPES OF PAPER	USES
CARTRIDGE PAPER	Expensive to buy Comes in different weights and sizes Best for small pieces of work, e.g. cards, water colour painting, paper sculpture, wax crayons
KITCHEN PAPER/NEWSPRINT	A thin off-white paper Useful for quick experimental paintings, pencil or crayon work
NEW ART PAPER	Thin but quite strong White Good for pencil, felt tip or crayons
SUGAR PAPER	Comes in different weights and colours Best for poster or powder colour Thin weight good for picture mounting Dark shades are good for oil pastels or chalks Sugar paper is also good for collage
CARD	Comes in different weights and colours Expensive but good for construction or 3D work Card from cereal packets etc. is just as effective if models are to be painted
TISSUE PAPER	Comes in squares, circles and sheets in a variety of different colours. Best used with white or light coloured sugar paper, being transparent Good for colour mixing activities when colour overlaps Easily torn or crumpled for textural effects
GUMMED PAPER	Comes in coloured shapes Good for collage if used with other materials
ACTIVITY PAPER	Hard surface paper in rich bright colours Suitable for paper sculpture, collages, chalks and pastels
COLLECTABLE PAPERS	Newspaper Wallpaper Colour magazines are good for collage Gift wrapping paper scraps Sweet papers (foil or coloured cellophane)

3. CHOOSING AND PREPARING PLAY ACTIVITIES

TOOLS THAT CAN BE USED FOR CREATIVE PLAY	
PENCILS	Pencils come in different thicknesses H is a normal writing pencil 2B, 4B, 6B etc. are soft The higher the number the softer the lead 2H, 4H, 6H are only suitable for adults It is important to use a soft pencil for drawing Very young children need thick pencils as they do not have the physical skills to hold a thin pencil
CHARCOAL	A soft drawing medium Smudges well (which may be frustrating for young children) Fixative can be used to stop it smudging
BIRO PENS	Good for line drawing and pattern
WAX CRAYONS	Can be used on wet paper
PASTELS	Soft thin chalks like board chalks Fine and provide a wide variety of colours Good for blending Can be mixed with water, applied with brush over top
PAINTS BLOCKS	Can be difficult to use Best to wet them half an hour before being used
POWDER COLOUR	Cheaper than poster colour Good if mixed in large quantities Careful mixing is important otherwise it is to thin or thick for children to use Mixing powder paint - use a yoghurt carton one quarter full of water to a carton of powder
POSTER COLOUR	Wide variety of bottled types and tubes. Kept in lidded pots. There is little waste. It can be thickened with PVA glue. It also makes it shine.
BRUSHES	Wide variety of thicknesses and lengths Children normally use sizes 4, 8, 10 Household paint brushes can be used for large pictures

┌───┐
— **Memory Jogger** —

Use the chart on page 156 to help you to answer
the questions.

1. What would you use the following papers for:
   a. Kitchen paper/newsprint
   b. Sugar paper
   c. Cartridge paper?
2. Name some papers that you could use for collage work.
3. What pencils are best for young children to use when drawing?
4. Name some tools that could be used for drawing.
5. How would you mix powder colour to make it thick enough for young children to use? (Try it and see if it works.)
└───┘

Preparing for an art activity

1. Make sure that the equipment and materials are ready to use before the activity begins. This should include painting aprons for the children.

2. Find somewhere safe for the finished work to dry.

3. Limit the materials that the children use, so that they are not confused too much by choice.

4. Make sure that the materials are attractively laid out for use.

5. If you are helping the child to learn a new skill for the first time, keep the materials simple e.g. do not give a child a thick piece of material to cut if they have not used scissors before.

6. Encourage a wider variety of materials when the child is more confident.

7. Children need time to experiment with the materials. Directed activities can be used to show the children new skills.

8. Check that the equipment is cared for when cleaning up after an activity i.e. brushes, paste, spreaders, tables etc.

9. Children's imagination can be stimulated in a number of different ways e.g. reading a book, a visit, a television programme, seasonal interests, nursery or class topics.

Dough

The sense of touch is an important way of exploring the world. If you watch young children when they are introduced to an object for the first time they will automatically want to touch, stroke and feel it. Play dough can help to develop the child's sense of touch.

Home made play dough is cheap and easy to make with children. Put it in a plastic bag or box and it will keep for a few weeks.

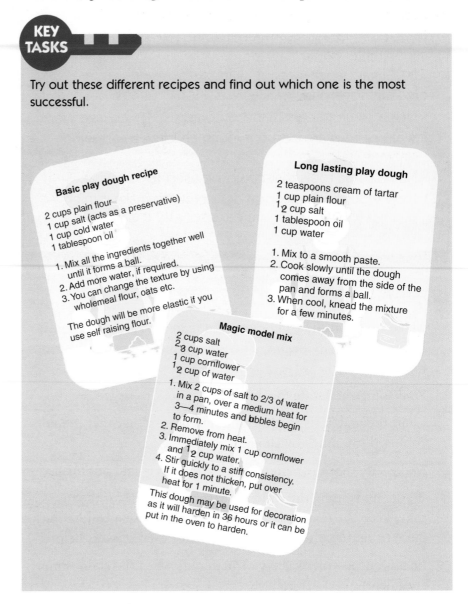

KEY TASKS

Try out these different recipes and find out which one is the most successful.

Basic play dough recipe

2 cups plain flour
1 cup salt (acts as a preservative)
1 cup cold water
1 tablespoon oil

1. Mix all the ingredients together well until it forms a ball.
2. Add more water, if required.
3. You can change the texture by using wholemeal flour, oats etc.

The dough will be more elastic if you use self raising flour.

Long lasting play dough

2 teaspoons cream of tartar
1 cup plain flour
1 2 cup salt
1 tablespoon oil
1 cup water

1. Mix to a smooth paste.
2. Cook slowly until the dough comes away from the side of the pan and forms a ball.
3. When cool, knead the mixture for a few minutes.

Magic model mix

2 cups salt
2 3 cup water
1 cup cornflower
1 2 cup of water

1. Mix 2 cups of salt to 2/3 of water in a pan, over a medium heat for 3—4 minutes and bubbles begin to form.
2. Remove from heat.
3. Immediately mix 1 cup cornflower and 1 2 cup water.
4. Stir quickly to a stiff consistency. If it does not thicken, put over heat for 1 minute.

This dough may be used for decoration as it will harden in 36 hours or it can be put in the oven to harden.

Clay

Clay allows children to explore texture, develop manipulative skills and to create a variety of different objects. When children are given clay for the first time they should be given the chance to experiment with it, rather than being told to make specific objects.

Clay should be soft enough to handle on its own. If you add water it makes it very slippery and difficult to handle.

Preparing children to work with clay

✳ The children must roll up their sleeves and put on aprons before they play with the clay.

* The table should have a surface that can be easily washed. If not, then you should cover the table with a sheet of plastic.
* Each child should be given a lump of clay to work with.
* Let the children feel the clay and 'work it' by pulling, pushing and poking it.
* Sometimes the children enjoy using different tools with the clay, e.g. a blunt knife, lolly pop sticks, cotton reels, spatulas, plastic moulds.
* When the children have finished make sure they wash their hands well.
* The clay should be stored in a polythene bag or in an airtight container.

Activities with clay

* Flatten a ball of clay with the hands, and see how many textures can be made with the hands only i.e. pinching, banging, pressing.
* Use different objects to make marks on the clay e.g. nail heads, scoring the surface with a comb.
* Roll the clay thinly and twist or plait the strands.
  Arrange the rolls of clay in spirals or overlaps.
  Make faces, buildings, animals etc. with the rolls of clay
* Make small pellets from the clay. They can be used to make beads for necklaces, decorations for tiles or pots.
* Make a pot or other small container from a lump of clay.
* Coil pots can be made from rolls of clay. This can be done with seven and eight year old children.

Imaginative play

Do you remember pretending to be a nurse or a teacher when you were young? This is one type of **imaginative** play.

We all enjoy dressing up. We put on special clothes for a wedding or a party. What we wear has an influence on how we behave. The fun of being someone else begins when a child is quite young.

Imaginative play is fun. Children love the feel of walking in long skirts with high heeled shoes or wearing a fire fighter's helmet on their head. It gives them the chance to practice skills that they will use when they are older, e.g. driving, steering, cooking, sorting. Being someone else gives a child the chance to separate reality from fantasy.

Imaginative play lets the child bring out into the open any anxieties or worries in a safe environment. They can live through experiences that have frightened or shocked them. Children can be angry or violent with their dolls without doing any harm.

What children learn from imaginative play

Social development
Sharing materials
Choosing roles
Negotiating with others
Acting out problems
Working with others

Language development
Using different language
in a variety of situations
Listening to other
children's ideas
Using correct language

Intellectual development
Trying out new ideas
Developing imagination
and creativity
Developing a sequence
of events
Remembering past
experiences
Predicting what might
happen next
Using objects to
represent other things
Matching and sorting
different equipment
Counting, sorting,
matching
Problem solving

Emotional development
Getting rid of frustrations
Fun
Act out difficult situations in a safe environment,
e.g. going into hospital for the first time

Physical development
Hand and eye co-
ordination
Fine manipulative skills,
e.g. fastening buttons
on the dressing up
clothes

Activities and equipment to encourage imaginative play

Home area

All child care settings should have a home area. The home area should have equipment that reflects the child's culture and other cultures.

* Where possible, the equipment should be the 'real thing'. However the children must be safe.
* Cups, cooking pots, cutlery, plates, trays.
* Cupboards to store the equipment. The children should be encouraged to put the equipment away themselves.
* Different sized dolls representing different cultures.
* Dressing up clothes.

✳ Furniture, e.g. table, chairs, bed.

✳ Kitchen equipment, e.g. cooker, sink, iron and ironing board.

✳ Magazines, newspapers, road maps, calendar, recipe books, note book, telephone and telephone directory.

The children can also be encouraged to make their own equipment, e.g. television.

Children in their own homes can create a home area under the dining room table or in a small corner of their bedroom.

Dressing up clothes

Children love dressing up.

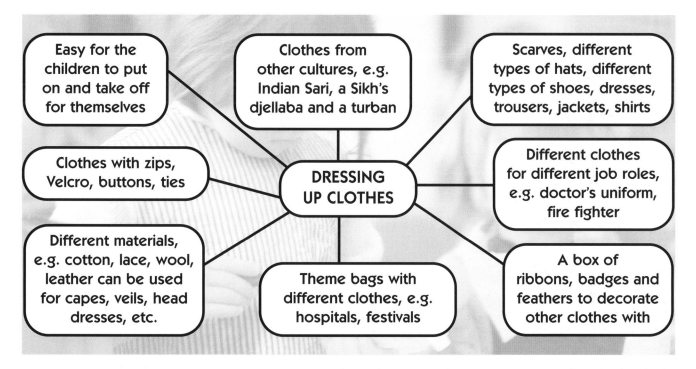

Easy for the children to put on and take off for themselves

Clothes from other cultures, e.g. Indian Sari, a Sikh's djellaba and a turban

Scarves, different types of hats, different types of shoes, dresses, trousers, jackets, shirts

Clothes with zips, Velcro, buttons, ties

DRESSING UP CLOTHES

Different clothes for different job roles, e.g. doctor's uniform, fire fighter

Different materials, e.g. cotton, lace, wool, leather can be used for capes, veils, head dresses, etc.

Theme bags with different clothes, e.g. hospitals, festivals

A box of ribbons, badges and feathers to decorate other clothes with

Puppets

Puppets can encourage imaginative play particularly for shy children and those who have speech difficulties.

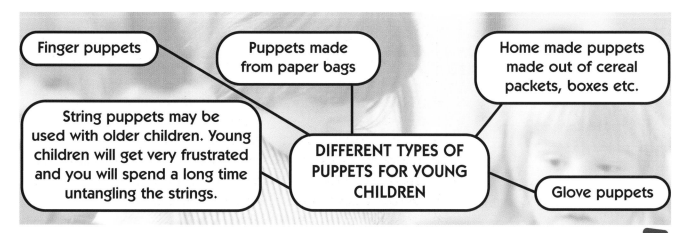

Finger puppets

Puppets made from paper bags

Home made puppets made out of cereal packets, boxes etc.

String puppets may be used with older children. Young children will get very frustrated and you will spend a long time untangling the strings.

DIFFERENT TYPES OF PUPPETS FOR YOUNG CHILDREN

Glove puppets

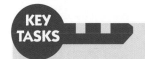

KEY TASKS

Make some hand puppets from paper bags or modelling materials. Take on the role of the puppet and make up a play. Do not write it down. Use your imagination.

The role of the adult in imaginative play

The adult must be very sensitive. The children will learn as they use the equipment. If the adult disturbs the child's play it can spoil the freshness of the play.

The adult must observe the children before joining in the play. They can then take on the role of a character in the play and ask questions or pose problems. This could improve the quality of the play.

Sand and water play

What children learn from sand and water play:

Intellectual development
Sorting materials
Remembering what has happened before
Repeating the activity
Adding new ideas
Discovering what sand and water can do
Concentrating on the activity
Scientific discoveries

Language development
Describing what has been done
Talking about the materials

Social development
Involving adults and other children in what has been discovered
Watching and working with others
Sharing materials

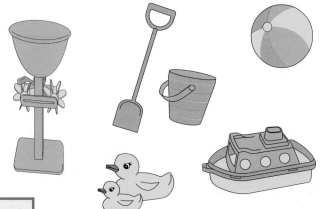

Physical development
Fine manipulative skills
Hand and eye coordination

Emotional development
Soothing
Fun
Calming

Sand play

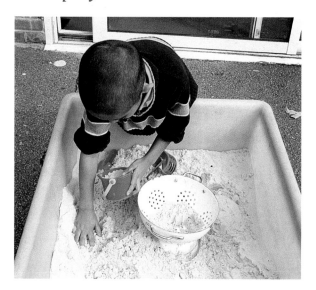

Children gain a great deal of pleasure and satisfaction from working with sand. It is an important sensory experience and can encourage children to learn new ideas and skills.

Sand reacts in different ways when it is dry, damp or very wet. Young children need to experience and compare all three textures.

Children can explore the sand with their hands or feet (in the sand pit). They can hold, pour and push the sand about or draw pictures with their fingers.

Sand play equipment

✳ Collection of spoons, scoops and spades of varying sizes
✳ Buckets
✳ Sand wheel and funnel
✳ Plastic and cardboard tubes
✳ Teapots, cups and jugs
✳ Various containers e.g. ice cream tubs
✳ Sieves including tea strainers, colanders, flowerpots
✳ Add pebbles, shells, gravel etc.
  and lots more!

KEY TASKS

① Visit a number of different shops that sell children's toys and equipment.

② Make a list of the toys or equipment that could be used by the children in their sand play.

③ Design a poster showing the different pieces of equipment and explain how the child may use them.

Water play

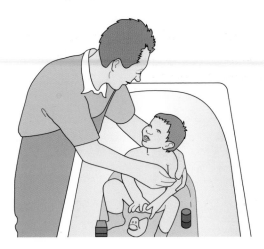

Water play begins when the child has their first bath and the carer gently splashes water over the new baby. The adult may talk or sing to the baby and smile while making eye contact.

When the child is old enough to sit up unaided, they can be supported on the kitchen floor with a small amount of tepid water. The baby can then pat it, run their fingers through it, wash itself with it and enjoy the soothing effect it can have.

The baby must never be left on their own when playing with water.

When the child is tall enough and steady enough on their feet to stand at the kitchen sink then they may 'do the washing up'. The adult may add washing detergent and the child's toys or doll's clothes may be added.

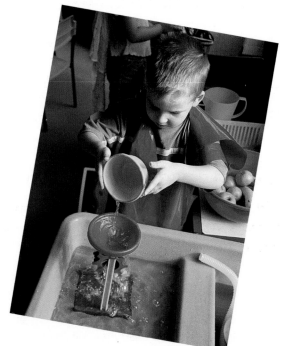

If the child is standing on a stool, always make sure that it is steady and not too high.

When the child is at nursery or play group, they will be given the opportunity to play with water in different ways; with other children and with different pieces of equipment.

Water play equipment

* Different sizes of funnels
* Different sizes and shapes of containers
* Different lengths and widths of hose
* Plastic bottles - some with holes in them
* Water mills and pumps
* Channels
* A collection of jugs, cups, scoops, spoons of varying sizes and lots more!

KEY TASKS

Visit a nursery or playgroup and watch a group of children working at the water tray for at least ten minutes.

* List the pieces of equipment that the children are using.

* Watch the children and describe what they do, e.g. do they talk to each other, how good is their concentration.

* What do you think the child/children might be learning?

* What protective clothing has been provided to make sure that the children keep as dry as possible?

Remember that the floor will get wet. Always dry it up before the child or adult walks on it.

The adult must observe the child carefully when they are playing with water particularly if they are playing in a paddling pool out of doors.

Construction play

Did you ever play with Lego when you were a child? This is perhaps the most popular piece of equipment that is used to encourage construction play.

What children learn from construction play

Physical development
Hand and eye co-ordination
Spatial awareness
Develop strength in fingers and hands
Discover different materials, e.g. textures, feeling holes

Intellectual development
Use different ideas to create structures
Copy design plans
Matching, sequencing
Problem solving
Invent own ideas
Use other children's ideas

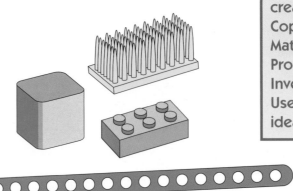

Language development
Talk about models
Explain how they have been made
Draw plans
Discuss plans with other children and adults
Listen to opinions of others

Emotional development
Sense of satisfaction when successful
Fun
Persist with the challenge
Learn to accept failure

Social development
Share equipment and space
Work with others
Take turns
Make something for someone else

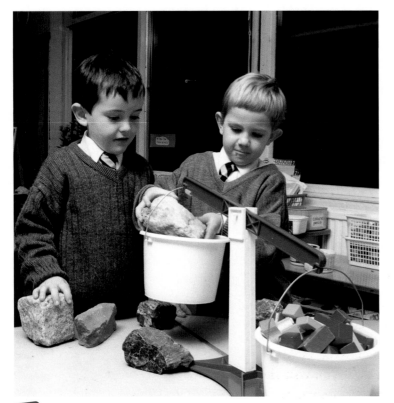

Equipment for Construction play

Provide a carpeted area with well organised, freely available materials. These could include:

* Meccano
* Stickle bricks
* Wooden blocks of different sizes
* Multilink
* Lego

The children will need lots of space and time to build their models.

Other equipment may be added to encourage imaginative play, e.g. cars, dinosaurs, miniature people.

Social play

Children learn when they play together. They find out how to share, take turns and co-operate with each other. They discover what kind of behaviour is expected in different situations, e.g. at home and in a restaurant. Friendships can develop during social play.

Playing games

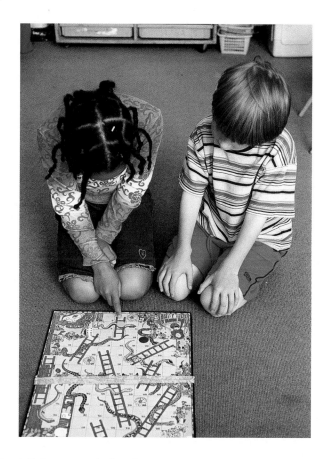

Playing a game with children can help them to:

✳ Learn how to keep rules and follow instructions
✳ Play together
✳ Have fun
✳ Cope with losing
✳ Solve problems
✳ Concentrate
✳ Learn new words and new concepts (ideas)

Table top games for different aged children

There is a wide range of table top games available for children and adults, e.g. dominoes, scrabble, lotto games, snakes and ladders.

Carry out a survey to find out the differences between table top games that are available for children and adults. If you visit shops remember to get permission from the manager before you start.

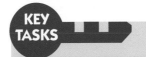

KEY TASKS

A group of three and four year-old children are about to play a lotto game. Sunita, Matthew and David look at the pictures and talk about them while Beth puts the board on the table. Sunita and David begin to argue over who is going to give the cards out. Bethany says, 'It's Matthew's turn because we promised him yesterday'. The children sit down at the table and Matthew collects all the playing cards together. Bethany calls out, 'Hurry up, Ben, we're waiting for you'. Ben leaves the cars he is playing with and joins the group. Matthew begins to give out the cards one by one, very carefully and deliberately. Matthew gets a bit confused between giving out the cards and filling up his own board. He cannot concentrate on both tasks at the same time.

An adult sees that Matthew is having difficulty and asks if she can give out the cards. The game continues with the adult's help and Ben wins. The adult says, 'Well done Ben. Give him a clap everyone'. Sunita says' It's not fair. I wanted to win'. The game goes on until everyone has put all the cards on the boards. The adult says well done to the children.

Write a short paragraph explaining:

a) What each child has learned from playing the game
b) What the adult did to help the children

Now complete the missing spaces using the words in the box below to help.

**intellectual   accepted   development   increases   valued   language
talk   instructions   esteem   social   participating   concentrate
questions   handle   emotional   hard   listening   praising   physical**

E............... d.................... is encouraged because the children all feel a............... and v............... as part of the s............... group. The children's ability to play the game i........... their self .... and helps them to feel emotionally satisfied.

Children accept that there has to be a winner. It can be h............... for children to accept that they cannot always win and the adult encourages them by p...........everyone so showing that p...........in the game is important.

I............. development is encouraged when the children look at the pictures. The ability to c................ is developed as they have to watch and think about what is happening.

L .... skills are also developed. They talk to each other, listen to i.......... and ask q...............

P............. skills can be developed when they are h............. the cards.

Table top games for children

1–2 years

Most children of this age like to play games on their own. They do not want to share or take turns. An adult can help the child begin to learn these skills. Simple matching and sorting games can be played.

2–3 years
Children are beginning to understand how to share and they will enjoy playing lotto games. They do not usually have the concentration or physical skills to play board games using counters, dice or small playing pieces.

3–5 years
By this stage most children are able to share, take turns and are beginning to understand how other children feel. They are able to follow simple rules and they can ask questions if they do not understand. Children begin to play games that involve dice and counters, providing they are not too small.

5–8 years
Older children can play a wide variety of table top games. They have a good understanding of how to take turns and follow rules. They particularly enjoy games with a purpose.

KEY TASKS

Design a poster, which shows the different types of table-top games that are available for children of different ages. Show the age of the child that each game is appropriate for and make notes on what the child can learn from the game.

Survey of table top games

Look at three different board or table top games and complete the chart below.

	1	2	3
① What age of children can play the game?			
② Does the game encourage winning and losing?			
③ How many children can play the game?			
④ Can the children play it on their own without getting help from adults?			
⑤ Are the rules complicated?			
⑥ Do the children have to take turns?			
⑦ Can children who have specific needs play the game?			
⑧ Which game do you like best and why?			

**KEY
TASKS**

Make a table top game for a small group of children. Before you begin
you will need to decide:

① What age the game will be for.

② How many children will be able to play the game.

③ What the rules of the game are.

④ How you can ensure that all children can play the game whatever
their individual needs.

⑤ What safety issues need to be considered.

Play the game with a small group of children. Write a short paragraph
about the success of your game.

Jigsaws

Tip it out ⟶ Force pieces into the ⟶ Try out
wrong place | different shapes
but they do not
know if it is right

↓

Begin to look at the
picture

Look at the shape of
each piece before
trying to put it into
the right place

↑

Begin to look for the ⟵ Do the jigsaw again ⟵ Listen to adult
straight edges | if they are successful | suggestions

It is satisfying especially
when it is finished

The child has to use
different ways of
getting it right

Encourages fine
manipulative skills

Learn to co-operate
with others

**How jigsaws help a
child to learn**

Learn to share with
others

Problem solving

Encourages
concentration and
patience

Learn about shape
and colour matching

Stories and rhymes

Why are books important for young children?

Books

✳ are interesting and can give pleasure
✳ can increase a child's general knowledge and vocabulary
✳ can help a child learn more about different cultures and
religions

✺ can help in the development of all aspects of the curriculum, e.g. mathematics, science, technology

✺ can help in the development of language and communication

✺ can allow children to experience frightening or new situations within a safe environment

✺ can help increase the child's concentration span.

What kind of books should we choose?

There are so many good books available that it is difficult knowing where to begin.

Start from a personal viewpoint. Do you like the story? Do you find it exciting? Is it sad or funny? Are you enthusiastic about it? If the book appeals to you then you will enjoy reading the story to the children and they are more likely to enjoy it too.

Young children like a wide range of different stories. They usually enjoy a book that has a clear beginning, middle and end. They enjoy simple, fast-moving, straightforward plots, especially with an obvious ending. They like stories about animals and ones that make them laugh.

All children should be provided with books, which reflect different cultures and religions.

KEY TASKS

Visit the children's section of your local library. Look at the books and find one that you like. Now answer the following questions.

✺ What age of children do you think would enjoy the book?

✺ Why did you choose the book? Give **three** different reasons.

✺ What do you think the children will learn from listening to the story?

AGE GROUP	WHAT TO LOOK FOR WHEN CHOOSING BOOKS
0–3 YEARS	Colourful bold pictures tough light able to be wiped Easy to handle rounded corners clear print Familiar objects 'bath, cloth, board and theme' books
3–5 YEARS	Simple plot central character gives a sense of security Repeated phrases predictable endings more print Pictures showing lots of action families, pets, familiar objects Funny books naughty children
5–8 YEARS	Imaginative stories stories from the past more print but smaller science fiction Longer stories that are more complex A range of different characters

Reading books to young children

Ten simple rules to follow when reading books to children

1. Be prepared. Read the book yourself before you read it to the children. You may have to do it more than once to make sure you know the story well.

2. Practise reading the story aloud.

3. Make sure the children can see the book and can hear you.

4. Tell the children the title of the book and who wrote it.

5. Use different tones of voice for different characters in the story and lots of expression

6. Speak clearly and not too fast. However you might want to talk quickly if you are reading an exciting part. Speak slowly if you want to emphasise something.

7. Practise holding the book so that the children can see the pictures.

8. Watch the children as you are reading the story.

9. Encourage the children to join in when there are repetitive parts to the story.

10. Ask questions to make sure that the children are listening. However, be careful that you do not spoil the story by asking too many questions.

Encouraging children to listen to the story

If you are well prepared and the book is suitable for the children

KEY TASKS

Choose a book that you think the children will enjoy or ask the children to choose one for you. Read it through several times so that you know the story well. Read the book to the children.

Write a short description of what happened. Your description should include:

* The title and author of the book

* The number of children you read the story to

* Where you read the story?

* What happened?

then it is likely that your story-telling session will be trouble free. However, some children find it difficult to listen and you will have to help them.

KEY TASKS

Grandma and Granddad

Here are grandma's spectacles
Here is grandma's hat
This is the way she folds her hands
And puts them in her lap.

Here are granddad's glasses
Here is granddad's hat
This is the way he folds his arm
And takes a little nap.

Source: unknown

A Little Rabbit

A little rabbit on a hill
Was bobbing up and down
His little tail was soft and white
His two long ears were brown.

But when he heard a tiny noise
His eyes were black as coal
His little whiskers trembled
And he scuttled down a hole.

Source: unknown

Children enjoy learning rhymes that have simple actions. What actions could you use for each of the rhymes above? Learn the rhyme off by heart and tell it to a child or small group of children using the actions that you have planned.

Some finger rhymes help children to learn about numbers.

One kitten two kittens three
    kittens four
Fast asleep on the kitchen floor
One miaow, two miaows, three
    miaows four
Wake the kittens on the floor.

With one squeak, two squeaks,
    three squeaks four
They chased the puppies out the
    door.

Source: unknown

Astronauts are ready
Everything is 'Go'
Instruments are ready
Time to countdown so
10 9 8 7 6 5 4 3 2 1
Zero
Blast off

Source: unknown

KEY TASKS

Find two finger rhymes that would be suitable for a three year-old child. Learn the words and the actions. Use the rhymes with a child you know well. Write a short paragraph about what happened and how the child reacted.

✹ Make sure that the children are comfortable and can see the book before you begin.

✹ If you know the child's name, mention their name as though they were part of the story.

✹ Make eye contact with the child who has lost concentration.

✹ Ask the child a question.

Music

Many people who work with young children do not provide music activities because they feel they are not musical themselves. You do not need to be musical to encourage children to enjoy music. All you need to know is what kind of equipment is suitable for young children and a lot of enthusiasm.

There are four different areas of music.

① Singing

② Playing

③ Listening

④ Moving

What can a child learn from music

Physical development
Hand and eye co-ordination
Control of different instruments
Use different parts of the body to move to music

Language development
Tell the difference between sounds

Intellectual development
Improve concentration
Listen to instructions
Copy sounds and rhythms
Remember different patterns and sequences of music
Remembering words of songs
Learn about other cultures

Social development
Turn taking
Sharing instruments with others
Being part of a group

Emotional development
Pleasure
Appreciate different sounds and moods
Sense of satisfaction when composing music

Singing

Choosing songs for young children:

* Try to choose a song that the children will enjoy. It may have funny words or good actions.
* Do not sing songs that are too long.
* If the children are very young, try to find songs that are repetitive and easy to learn.
* Use actions if you can.
* Avoid songs that are too high to sing.
* Children like singing songs they know well.

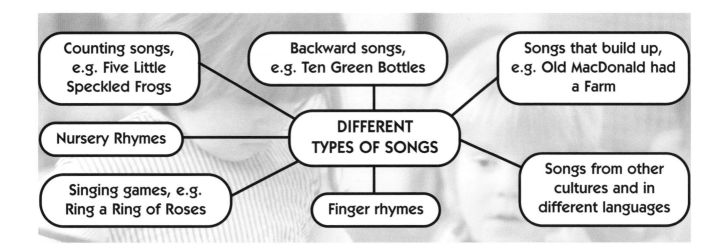

Counting songs, e.g. Five Little Speckled Frogs

Backward songs, e.g. Ten Green Bottles

Songs that build up, e.g. Old MacDonald had a Farm

Nursery Rhymes

DIFFERENT TYPES OF SONGS

Songs from other cultures and in different languages

Singing games, e.g. Ring a Ring of Roses

Finger rhymes

Playing

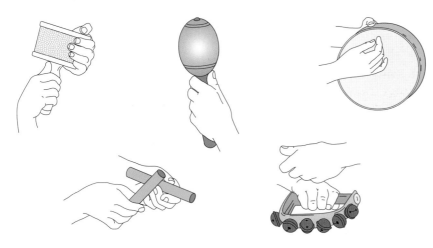

How many instruments do you know?

Listening

Children need to be able to listen to enjoy music and develop language skills. The child needs to learn to:

* ✹ concentrate
* ✹ understand what he/she is listening to
* ✹ remember what he/she has heard.

Listening games

Body sounds

Different parts of our body can make different sounds. Encourage the children to find out what sound their hands can make, e.g. clap, snap, click

What sounds do their feet make, e.g. stamping, running on different surfaces, hopping

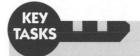

Use different body sounds to accompany this poem.

It's raining, it's pouring
The old man is snoring
He went to bed and he bumped his head
And could not get up in the morning.

Try this activity with a group of children.

Sounds around us

Encourage the children to listen to the sounds around them. Can they hear the birds, traffic, wind etc? Can they use different instruments to make them sound like the birds, traffic etc?

Playing

When you give instruments to young children it is very important to give them time to play freely with them. Always work with a small group of children. If you have a big group they will make a lot of noise and they will be difficult to manage.

Here comes the band

Use a tape of marching music. Let the children choose an instrument and play along with the tape. Choose a tape that has a very steady beat and is lively.

Moving

Children love moving to music from a very young age.

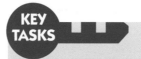

Watch a toddler when a music tape is being played. What happens?

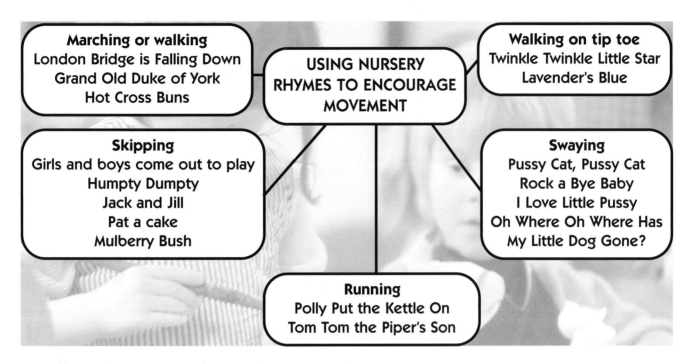

You may not know all these rhymes but you can add you own ones. Try to find rhymes from other cultures.

4. WHAT THE ADULT DOES WHEN THE CHILD IS PLAYING

When children are playing, you should:

* Watch them to make sure they are safe.
* Watch carefully and think about what you have learned about how children grow and develop.
* Join in with the children but do not impose your ideas on them.
* Become a character. If the children are playing in the home area you must wait to be invited in and you should take on an appropriate role. If you do not do this, the children's play will stop.
* Ask questions that will encourage the children to give you more than one word answers.
* Answer questions.
* Help to improve their skills, e.g. if a child is having difficulty using a pair of scissors you may give them some suggestions on how to hold the paper or the scissors.
* Play with the child.
* Let them have time on their own to explore a new toy and find out what it can do. Later on, you can offer the child more challenging experiences.
* Encourage them during their play.

When the children have finished playing it is important to talk to your work place supervisor about what you have seen. He/she can then make sure that the activities that are available for the children the next day, will help to improve their skills.

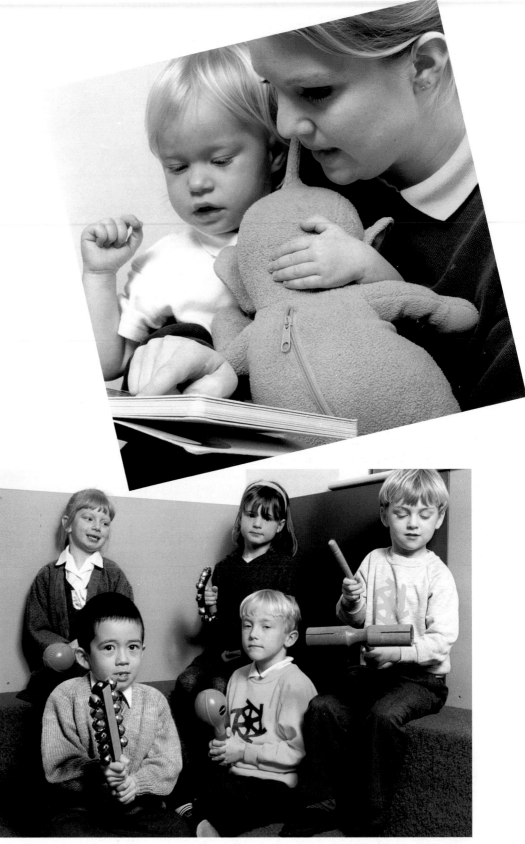

TEST YOURSELF

① Find the eight different types of play

C	O	N	S	T	R	U	C	T	I	O	N
X	R	S	H	E	L	O	K	T	F	D	C
O	U	E	T	C	F	G	N	M	I	U	D
V	B	A	A	P	L	K	J	H	G	F	W
L	W	V	B	T	S	D	E	W	N	B	V
A	H	G	V	B	I	G	V	C	X	I	N
C	B	Y	U	T	R	V	K	M	J	R	D
I	S	D	W	Q	I	B	E	O	U	Y	Z
S	O	C	I	A	L	B	F	K	H	N	E
Y	F	G	H	S	W	Q	D	N	A	S	P
H	B	Y	U	T	F	K	S	A	P	M	B
P	E	V	I	T	A	N	I	G	A	M	I

② A three year-old child is playing with the telephone in the home area. What type of play is this?

③ How can creative play promote the social and emotional development of the child? Give **three** reasons.

④ It is a beautiful day and the staff have decided to take the equipment outside. They are working on a pirate theme and so they take out planks, barrels, rubber tyres and the climbing frame.

    a) What type of play could the children be involved in?
    b) How can this type of play encourage the physical and intellectual development of the children?

⑤ Bricks, lego, sticklebricks and meccano are examples of equipment used to encourage a type of play. Name this type of play.

⑥ A child care worker has put out some paper, paints and different shaped bricks and cotton reels. The child care worker watched the children as they used the materials. Joan used the cotton reel, a brick and one colour of paint only. She started to make a picture of a house. She used the edge of the brick to make the lines for the walls of the house. She then used the cotton reels to print the windows.

How can this type of play help Joan's language and physical development?

⑦ Name **three** natural materials that a child could play with.

⑧ Name **four** areas of music that a child can take part in.

⑨ What should the adult do when children are playing? Describe **four** examples.

⑩ What types of books would you give to:

a) a baby
b) a three year-old child
c) a five year-old child?

And Finally

If you are reading this page, then it means that you have almost finished your course. Well done! Why not find out how much you know about caring for young children.

Test yourself for the last time.

① What does gross motor skills mean? Give **two** examples.
  What does fine manipulative skills mean? Give **two** examples.

  4 marks

② Name the main nutrients that are found in food.

  P _ _ _ _ _ _
  I _ _
  C _ _ _ _ _ _ _ _ _
  M _ _ _ _ _ _
  F _ _ _ _ _
  V _ _ _ _ _ _ _
  F _ _

  7 marks

③ Describe **three** ways of keeping food safe in the refrigerator.

  6 marks

④ Food labels have the following terms on them. What do they mean?
  a 'use by' date
  b 'best before' date.

  4 marks

⑤ Explain where raw meat should be stored in the refrigerator. Give **three** reasons for your answer.

  3 marks

⑥ Name **three** different types of play that you would see in the nursery.

  3 marks

⑦ What does 'social development' mean?   **2 marks**

⑧ What would you do if a three year-old child was burnt on the hand?

  3 marks

⑨ Name **two** different types of child abuse.   **2 marks**

⑩ What would you do if you thought a child in the nursery was being abused?

3 marks

⑪ Why are children sometimes difficult to manage? Give **three** reasons.

3 marks

⑫ Why do adults sometimes find it difficult to manage children? Give **three** reasons.

3 marks

⑬ What should the adult do when children are playing? Give **five** examples.

10 marks

⑭ Match the type of social play to the correct name.

Two children are playing with the same toys but are not playing together.	Associative play
The child is standing on her own watching another group of children playing.	Parallel play
A group of children are playing together on the same task.	Solitary play
A child is playing on its own.	Co-operative play

4 marks

⑮ What are the basic needs of a child? Give **three** examples.

3 marks

Total 60 marks

How well did you do?

✳ To get a pass you would need to score between **30 and 35** marks.

✳ To get a merit you would need to score between **36 and 47** marks.

✳ To get a distinction you would need to score **48** marks or above.

Useful Addresses

The National Early Years Network
77 Holloway Road
London
N7 8JZ

The National Society for the Prevention for Cruelty to Children (NSPCC)
3 Gilmour Close
Beaumont Leys
Leicester
LE4 1EZ

For free information and support on:

How to stop smoking contact Smokeline
on 0800 84 84 84

How to stop drug abuse contact the National
Drugs Helpline on 0800 77 66 00

Re-Solv
The Society for the Prevention of Solvent and Volatile Substance Abuse
30 High Street
Stone
Staffordshire
ST15 8AW
National Freephone Helpline0808 800 2345
www.re-solv.org

British Allergic Foundation
St Bartholomew's Hospital
West Smithfield
London
EC1A 7BE

The Hyperactive Children's Support Group
71 Whyke Lane
Chichester
West Sussex
PO19 2LD (send a SAE)

The Royal Society for the Prevention of Accidents
Edgbaston Park
353 Bristol Road
Edgbaston
Birmingham
B5 7ST
www.rospa.org.uk

The Child Accident Prevention Trust (CAPT)
Clerks Court
18–20 Farringdon Lane
London
EC1R 3AU

Index